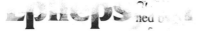

Clinical Practice
A Case Study Approach

Epilepsy in Clinical Practice
A Case Study Approach

Andrew N. Wilner, MD, FACP
Author of *Epilepsy: 199 Answers*

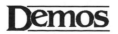

Demos Medical Publishing, Inc., 386 Park Avenue South, New York, New York 10016

Library of Congress Cataloging-in-Publication Data

Wilner, Andrew N.
    Epilepsy in clinical practice : a case study approach / Andrew N. Wilner.
        p. ; cm.
    Includes bibliographical references and index.
    ISBN 1-888799-34-X (alk. paper)
   1. Epilepsy—Case studies.
    [DNLM: 1. Epilepsy—Case Report. 2. Clinical Medicine—methods. WL 385 W744e 2000] I. Title.
   RC372.W554 2000
616.8′5309—dc21   00–064407

Made in the United States of America

Dedication

To my brothers, David and Matthew,
who inspire excellence while enforcing humility

Acknowledgments

Many thanks to my colleagues in the epilepsy community for sharing their knowledge and enthusiasm. A number of individuals graciously volunteered ideas or reviewed parts of the manuscript; Selim Benbadis, Dietrich Blumer, Lisa Breault, Maryann Brinley, Bruce Ehrenberg, Nancy Foldvary, Adelaide Hebert, Randy Kozel, Ilo Leppik, Sharon Parnes, Michele Sammaritano, Jeremy Slater, Marie-Helene St. Hilaire, Carmela Vittorio, H. Steve White, and Elaine Wyllie. Their comments enhanced the text and served as encouragement when the goal of completing this manuscript seemed unobtainable. Clearly, any inaccuracies are my own.

The Epilepsy Foundation, International Bureau for Epilepsy (IBE), and International League Against Epilepsy (ILAE) provided valuable information. In particular, Caroline Gallagher and Ann Little at the IBE and Irene Kujath at the ILAE were extraordinarily helpful.

Special thanks to my publisher, Dr. Diana M. Schneider, for her patience in helping me transform another challenging idea into a tangible reality.

Preface

More than 2 million Americans suffer from seizures. Each year, almost 200,000 people experience a seizure for the first time and approximately 100,000 require hospital admissions. The majority of these patients receive care from primary care physicians and general neurologists.

Epilepsy in Clinical Practice: A Case Study Approach highlights dramatic diagnostic and therapeutic advances that impact the medical care of patients with epilepsy. Computerized imaging studies, new and improved medications, refined brain surgery techniques, increased experience with the ketogenic diet, and the Food and Drug Administration approval of the vagal nerve stimulator have elevated the state of the art. Medical decision making has correspondingly increased in complexity. The primary goal of this book is to lend clarity and confidence to the practical management of patients with seizures.

This book represents one epileptologist's approach to the considerations and complications encountered when caring for patients with epilepsy. It's one thing to study a textbook about epilepsy, quite another to confront a patient with ill-defined symptoms and determine the best treatment. Ferreting out from the history what is important and what is extraneous, discerning the neurologic from the histrionic, and arriving at a diagnosis are among the most difficult challenges that face the physician. Once armed with a diagnosis, multiple treatment options exist. Choices must be individualized and patients educated in order for them to fruitfully participate in choosing appropriate diagnostic and treatment paths.

A dozen clinical cases drawn from my practice are presented for discussion, much as they would be during ward rounds. I struggled to find a compromise between short, pithy answers that respond to management questions and long didactic ones that delve deeper into the topic. My solution was to provide two answers, one "short," one "long." Sometimes all one wishes to read is a quick affirmation to a question. This answer appears immediately after the question. If more explication is desired, one can grapple with the longer answer that follows.

All recommendations are my own. They are based on my internship at the Long Beach Veterans Hospital, internal medicine residency at Los Angeles County Hospital, neurology residency at McGill, fellowship training at the Montreal Neurological Institute, six years as director of a comprehensive epilepsy program, a stint at an academic medical center, and personal experience treating more than a thousand patients with seizures.

Epilepsy in Clinical Practice does not pretend to be all-inclusive and exhaustive, but rather clear and accessible. For example, an understanding of the international classifications of seizures and epilepsy syndromes has become a fundamental requirement for successful patient management. For most users, these classifications are complex and cumbersome. Consequently, I have presented them in a condensed, simplified form (see Resources A and B). For the purist who requires the original, or for the student who has mastered the basics, the complete versions of these classifications can be found in references provided in the bibliography.

For easy accessibility, I have relied heavily on the Resources section. Tables, charts, and checklists respond to frequently asked questions. It includes Web sites for physicians and patients, state driving regulations, summer camps for children with epilepsy, local affiliates of the Epilepsy Foundation, chapters of the International League Against Epilepsy, contact telephone numbers for pharmaceutical companies, and numerous other resources.

The glossaries of acronyms and terms will facilitate communication between the generalist and the specialist, and are meant to supplement medical dictionaries. Neurology consultations, magnetic resonance imaging (MRI), and electroencephalogram (EEG) reports have a language all their own. For example, what is meant when the epileptologist suggests that seizures may be due to "pyknolepsy" or JME? A special section on understanding EEG jargon is also included (see Resource Z). Of course, there is no substitute for actually speaking to the report's author, but in today's busy practice setting, time for conversation does not always exist.

Information in the tables has been customized to correspond to my clinical experience. Dosing of antiepileptic drugs (AEDs) may vary somewhat from the *Physician's Desk Reference* (PDR). For example, the PDR lists 2 grams as the limit for Mysoline dose in adults. I rarely use more than 750 mg and have never seen a patient taking 2 grams. The usual adult dose listed in my table is 500–1500 mg.

I hope that this book will enhance the care of patients with epilepsy. It is written for general neurologists, primary care physicians, residents, medical students, physician assistants, pharmacists, nurses, social workers, and others. When used as directed, it should provide a mix of useful information and modest entertainment for those who strive to help patients with epilepsy.

Foreword

I am pleased to recommend this text to neurologists and other physicians who treat patients with epilepsy. Dr. Wilner has used his clinical experience in treating these patients and presents this material in a manner that covers the important aspects of managing the many problems that face both these patients and their treating physicians. Physicians will find it a thoughtful and helpful resource in their daily management of patients.

Dr. Wilner has divided his book into twelve chapters that cover various clinical scenarios encountered by physicians and their patients, including the first seizure, intractable epilepsy, stopping medications, epilepsy and pregnancy, allergic reactions, and other common problems encountered in epilepsy management.

Dr. Wilner uses clinical situations involving specific patients to introduce clinical problems, explore them, and discuss them in terms of clinical approaches, solutions, and overall patient management. He effectively uses these clinical situations to illustrate the many questions physicians encounter in their practice and brings together information that is critical to the thoughtful management of the patient with epilepsy. He demonstrates a considerate and empathetic approach to these patients.

The physician who has questions concerning how to manage specific problems such as the first seizure, the female patient who wants to become pregnant, the patients who fails medications, the patient who goes into status epilepticus will find an easy-to-read common-sense approach to these situations.

In addition to the clinical management of common problems encountered in caring for patients with epilepsy, the book contains an extensive section on resources that are available to physicians and patients, an excellent glossary of acronyms and terms, and selected references.

B.J. Wilder, M.D.

Table of Contents

Answered Questions

Chapter 3

Stopping Antiepileptic Medications

Chapter 4

Epilepsy and Medications

Chapter 5

Epilepsy and Pregnancy

Chapter 6

Rash!

Chapter 7

Epilepsy and Psychiatric Disorders

Chapter 8

Epilepsy in the Elderly

Chapter 9

Seizures and Alcohol

Chapter 10

Generalized Convulsive Status Epilepticus

Chapter 11

Nonepileptic Seizures

Chapter 12

Alternative Therapy

1

The First Seizure

Sandra is a 34-year-old single mother who awoke Saturday morning with a strange light-headedness. She waited on the edge of the bed for a few minutes until the feeling went away. Then she took a shower and got dressed. After eating breakfast, she found herself lying on the kitchen floor, her blouse splattered with scrambled eggs and a shattered coffee cup next to her. She didn't know what happened but got up and felt all right. She wasn't tired and had no headache.

About three in the afternoon, she remembers her 7-year-old daughter screaming at her to wake up. Sandra had fallen on the living room carpet. Her forehead throbbed where she had struck it on the coffee table, and her tongue hurt. Her daughter called 911, and they went to the hospital. Her mind felt foggy for the next two days.

When I saw Sandra in my office a week later, she told me she had never had similar episodes. There was no history of febrile seizures, myoclonic jerks, encephalitis, or meningitis. She never had unexplained spells during sleep. She denied any olfactory, auditory, or visual auras. She knew of a first cousin and a second cousin with epilepsy.

Gestation was complicated by diethylstilbestrol. Birth was premature. She weighed five pounds. Development was normal.

Both buttocks were severely scalded when she fell against a hot radiator as a baby. At the age of four, she was thrown off her bicycle and hit her head on the curb. She was unconscious for several minutes.

Sandra had gestational diabetes during her pregnancy. She had right eyelid surgery for congenital ptosis. She also had surgery on her left foot and a cholecystectomy.

Sandra has always had a nervous stomach. In college she developed an eating disorder that never really went away. The school psychologist told her she had anorexia nervosa. She weighed only 90 pounds during her sophomore year. She takes clonazepam for anxiety and mirtazapine for depression. She is allergic to codeine and hydrocodone.

Sandra married 10 years ago and dropped out of school before completing her senior year of college. Her husband left her six months ago, and she doesn't know where he is. She is unable to pay her bills and is looking for a job. She worries about providing for her daughter and doesn't sleep well.

She takes her medication regularly but missed one dose of clonazepam on the day she had the spells. A psychiatrist prescribed mirtazapine one month ago for depression and to help her gain weight. Her menstrual periods have been irregular and infrequent. She doesn't smoke, drink, or abuse drugs.

Sandra was a thin, healthy appearing young woman who weighed 100 pounds. She had a reticulated scar pattern on both buttocks. Neurologic examination revealed a mild ptosis on the right, but her vision was otherwise normal. Computed axial tomography scan without contrast, which was performed in the emergency room, suggested generalized atrophy.

Questions

1. Is it likely for Sandra to develop epilepsy at her age?

No.

Epilepsy is a disorder that is characterized by recurrent seizures. Seizures are clinical events caused by abnormal paroxysmal discharges of neurons that appear as spike and wave on the electroencephalogram (EEG). Symptoms depend on the cortical localization of the epileptic activity. For example, a temporal lobe focus may produce an epigastric aura; a frontal lobe seizure, motor movement; and an occipital lobe focus, flashing lights. Seizures that are provoked by a clear precipitant such as cocaine, alcohol withdrawal, or an electrolyte abnormality are not considered epilepsy.

In order to discern the etiology of a patient's seizures, one must begin with the age of onset. Congenital abnormalities are often responsible for seizures that begin in infancy. Epilepsy presenting in the elderly (see Chapter 8) usually results from cerebrovascular disease or brain tumors.

Sandra is 34 years old. New-onset epilepsy occurs more frequently in childhood and old age than in the middle adult years. Sandra is too old to have a congenital cause and relatively young for cerebrovascular disease. Numerous other possible etiologies, including head trauma, infection, vascular malformations, and neurodegenerative disease, remain.

Magnetic resonance imaging (MRI) has improved our diagnostic ability, revealing cases of mesial temporal sclerosis (MTS) and neuronal migration disorders with amazing clarity. But even after a comprehensive neurologic evaluation, the etiology of more than 50 percent of epilepsy cases remains unknown. These cases are termed "idiopathic" or "cryptogenic." Idiopathic cases are presumed to have a genetic basis, whereas cryptogenic epilepsy has a yet-to-be-discovered underlying lesion. Because Sandra presents at a relatively unusual age for new-onset epilepsy, one must also consider that these spells represent a medical or psychological disorder other than epilepsy (see Chapter 11).

2. Does Sandra have any risk factors for epilepsy?

Yes.

The patient's early history must be probed. Was gestation complicated by maternal infection with a TORCH (toxoplasmosis, rubella, cytomegalovirus, or herpes) infection? These congenital infections typically produce neonatal seizures. Was delivery difficult? Was the baby breech or blue? Were the Apgar scores low? Sandra was born with congenital ptosis. Was this related to birth trauma?

Details of early life are often sketchy in adult patients. School performance is a good objective measure of neurologic abilities. It is unlikely that Sandra had a congenital infection or has cerebral malformations, such as polymicrogyria, heterotopias, or lissencephaly, because she successfully completed three years of college.

She did strike her head at the time of her bicycle accident. Most active children suffer minor head injuries without neurologic sequelae. A head injury without loss of consciousness rarely constitutes a risk factor for epilepsy. The longer the interval from the accident to the seizure, the less likely it is that the head injury is responsible. Loss of consciousness or, more important, hospitalization, suggests a more severe head injury. Prolonged unconsciousness or amnesia, subdural hematoma, or brain hemorrhage characterize severe head trauma, which predisposes to epileptic seizures.

Sandra's head injury occurred 30 years ago, and she has been asymptomatic in the interim. Consequently, her head injury at age 4 is not likely to be related to her current seizures.

Is there a history of encephalitis or meningitis? These infections not only cause acute seizures, but also may be responsible for lifelong epilepsy. The risk of epilepsy increases five times after one has had bacterial meningitis and 10 times after an episode of viral encephalitis.

Sandra reports a history of epilepsy in two cousins. A family history of epilepsy is an important risk factor. More than 50 years ago, William Lennox pioneered the study of epilepsy genetics by compiling data on more than 4,000 patients. An obvious mendelian pattern of inheritance failed to emerge. Lennox proposed that both hereditary and acquired factors interact to produce epilepsy. This theory remains current today.

Genes have been identified for a number of different types of epilepsy: autosomal dominant nocturnal frontal lobe epilepsy, benign familial neonatal convulsions, benign familial infantile convulsions, familial temporal lobe epilepsy, and two autosomal recessive progressive myoclonic epilepsies—Unverricht-Lundborg disease and Batten disease. Maternally inherited mitochondrial encephalomyopathies have also been identified. However, all of these types of epilepsy are relatively uncommon.

A single autosomal gene cannot explain the most common genetic epilepsies. They display "complex" inheritance, which results from contributions of multiple genes combined with environmental interactions. Both childhood absence epilepsy and juvenile myoclonic epilepsy run in families and have complex inheritance patterns. Age-dependent penetrance is another feature of the genetic epilepsies.

Despite rapid advances in the field of epilepsy and molecular genetics, there is no commercial genetic test to aid the practitioner in the diagnosis of epilepsy. The fact that Sandra has two family members with seizures suggests that she may have a genetic epilepsy with complex inheritance and relatively late penetrance.

3. Did Sandra really have seizures?

I think so.

Sandra had three unexplained events. She awoke with a unique light-headed feeling. She may have been presyncopal, but the sensation lasted several minutes. The feeling may have been the residual of a partial complex seizure in her sleep. Partial seizures are the most common seizure type in adult-onset epilepsy, representing more than 70 percent of cases (see Resource A for Seizure Classification).

During breakfast, Sandra lost consciousness and awoke on the floor. She dropped her food and broke a cup, which suggests that the spell came on without warning. She does not remember what happened. Unfortunately, there was no witness to provide details of the event. The event may have been syncopal, because she did not complain of postictal headache or fatigue. On the other hand, there were no warning symptoms of malaise or light-headedness, which suggests that the event may have been a seizure. She may even have experienced an epileptic aura, but she cannot remember it.

Sandra again awoke on the floor in the afternoon, this time with a tongue laceration. Tongue biting can occur in syncope, but it is much more suggestive of a convulsion. She also had a significant amount of mental cloudiness for two days after the episode, probably representing postictal confusion. The most likely diagnosis at this point appears to be a localization-related epilepsy that presented with a partial complex seizure during sleep followed by two partial onset seizures evolving to convulsions. It appears that Sandra had three seizures in one day.

Many diseases imitate epilepsy. Syncope is the most common diagnosis confused with seizures. Sandra has no history of palpitations or shortness of breath to suggest cardiac disease. However, given her history of anorexia, an electrolyte imbalance such as hypokalemia might have precipitated a cardiac arrhythmia. An electrolyte panel and an electrocardiogram should be part of Sandra's emergency room (ER) evaluation. If any abnormalities appear, a Holter monitor would provide more information.

A hypoglycemic episode is another possibility. However, Sandra was eating at the time of her second spell and was unlikely to be sufficiently hypoglycemic to lose consciousness.

Transient ischemic attacks rarely present with loss of consciousness. A migraine aura could have caused her strange feeling upon awakening, but migraine is unlikely to account for the two later spells.

Sandra and her daughter were abandoned by her husband of 10 years. She is depressed and unemployed. The spells may represent conversion disorder, panic attacks, or even malingering.

4. Are these really new-onset seizures?

Maybe not.

Because the age of onset is so critical to the etiology of the seizure disorder, one must determine when the first seizure occurred. In addition, decisions about treatment focus on the likelihood of recurrence. If Sandra has a history of seizures, we are currently evaluating recurrent seizures, not new-onset seizures.

Sandra had an unfortunate, serious burn as an infant. Accidents happen, but one wonders if this wasn't a result of abuse or possibly an infantile convulsion that caused her to land on the radiator. She also had a bicycle accident with loss of consciousness. One could speculate that an absence or partial complex seizure caused the bicycle accident. A stronger case could be made for undiagnosed childhood epilepsy if there were more of these "accidents." Sandra denies staring spells, myoclonic jerks, or other unexplained episodes such as waking up on the floor next to her bed or not remembering how she arrived in a certain room in her house. There is no convincing evidence to suggest that Sandra ever had seizures before Saturday.

5. Could Sandra have seizures but not epilepsy?

Yes.

The important diagnostic issue is whether these seizures were spontaneous or provoked. If there is a clear precipitant for Sandra's seizures, one that could potentially be corrected or avoided in the future, these seizures do not constitute epilepsy. Rather than treatment with an antiepileptic medication, correction of the underlying cause is necessary. Patients commonly present to the ER with provoked seizures or develop them as inpatients concurrent with serious medical illness.

In the outpatient setting, metabolic disorders are responsible for seizures in less than 10 percent of cases. Glucose abnormalities are the most common metabolic problems. Hypoglycemia usually is due to insulin or oral hypoglycemic agents.

Hospital inpatients often have seizures related to electrolyte disorders. Hyponatremia (115 meq/l) affects 2.5 percent of hospitalized patients and can cause seizures (see Chapter 8). Hyponatremia must be corrected cautiously to avoid central pontine myelinolysis.

Severe hypocalcemia, hypomagnesemia, and hypophosphatemia can all cause seizures. Patients with hypoparathyroidism and associated hypocalcemia often have seizures. Convulsions occur in 25 percent of patients with hypothyroidism and myxedema coma. I remember only one patient who had seizures associated with hyperthyroidism. Once his thyroiditis was corrected, he did not require long-term therapy with antiepileptic drugs (AEDs). Hyperthyroidism is rarely a cause of seizures.

Seizures in patients with renal failure may be related to dialysis dysequilibrium syndrome (DDS), antibiotic toxicity, or uremic encephalopathy. Transplant patients may have intracerebral infections or primary central nervous system (CNS) lymphoma as an underlying etiology of seizures.

Seizures related to anoxia are commonly seen in the intensive care unit. They often are due to cardiac arrest, but other causes, such as carbon monoxide poisoning, near-drowning, near-hanging, respiratory failure, and complications of anesthesia, may be responsible. These seizures respond poorly to AEDs.

Sandra had been well until the time of her seizures. She was afebrile in the ER. Consequently, a CNS infection, such as meningitis, encephalitis, brain abscess, or parasite, seems unlikely.

Although her weight loss has been attributed to anorexia, celiac disease, ulcerative colitis, and Crohn's disease are all associated with an increased incidence of seizures. Patients with alcohol withdrawal (see Chapter 9) and hepatic encephalopathy have an increased incidence of seizures.

Recreational drugs must be considered as a cause of new-onset seizures in the young adult population. Amphetamines, cocaine, heroin, and phencyclidine all can cause seizures. A drug screen in the ER should be performed as part of the assessment of new-onset seizures.

Prescription drugs can also be epileptogenic. Tricyclic antidepressants (TCAs) are the most common offenders, with seizures occurring in approximately 1 percent of patients who take these medications. In general, selective serotonin reuptake inhibitors (SSRIs) are less epileptogenic than TCAs (see Chapter 7). Sandra began taking the antidepressant mirtazapine a month ago. Her psychiatrist chose this drug because one of its side effects is weight gain, which would be beneficial in Sandra's case. Mirtazapine can precipitate seizures in 1 of 1,000 patients. Coupled with other factors, such as Sandra's sleep deprivation and her missed clonazepam dose, mirtazapine may have contributed to her flurry of seizures.

6. Which definitive tests can determine whether Sandra's spells were epileptic?

None.

Epilepsy is a clinical diagnosis. The only sure way to ascertain that a spell is epileptic is to record the EEG simultaneously with the clinical event. This sometimes occurs fortuitously during routine EEG tracings, but it is more likely to happen during outpatient or inpatient monitoring with video-EEG equipment.

However, certain patterns on the EEG suggest epilepsy syndromes (see Resource Z). Definite spikes or spike and wave are rare in the normal population and their presence increases the likelihood of an epileptic disorder. Sharp waves are less definitive than spikes, but they also point to epilepsy.

A routine EEG records 20 minutes of brain waves. Routine EEGs capture a spike or sharp wave in approximately one half of patients with epilepsy. A sleep-deprived EEG or prolonged EEG significantly increases the yield. A prolonged EEG may also detect subclinical seizures.

Of course, even definite epileptic seizures recorded on the EEG do not establish that a *prior* spell was epileptic. Patients can have both epilepsy and syncope, or other diagnoses. The event in question may have been unrelated to the EEG findings.

Sandra's first EEG revealed very tiny bitemporal spikes and sharp waves. I interpreted these as benign variants known as small sharp spikes (SSS) of sleep. There was also excessive beta activity, which I attributed to her clonazepam, which is a benzodiazepine. A second EEG can improve the yield, so I ordered another. This one showed similar bitemporal spikes and sharp waves suggestive of SSS, as well as excessive beta activity. In addition, there were two brief bursts of sharp waves mixed with spikes. I thought these probably were epileptic, but they were so rare that I wondered whether they might be artifacts. Like any test, the EEG can be inconclusive. I thought the second EEG represented epileptic activity, but I wasn't sure.

Additional diagnostic tests of value are imaging studies. I am often asked which is better for diagnosing seizures—a computed axial tomography (CAT) scan or an MRI study? The answer really depends on the setting. In the ER, there very often is a question of head trauma with skull fracture or brain hemorrhage. The CAT scan is superior to MRI for these indications, can be obtained more quickly, and costs less.

However, MRI is preferred if trauma and blood are not high on the list of considerations, because this technology provides better visualization of the soft tissues and increases the likelihood of finding abnormalities in the cerebral cortex. Mesial temporal sclerosis (MTS) and neuronal migration disorders can be invisible on CAT scans, but are well appreciated on MRI. In a study of chronic epilepsy patients, the likelihood of finding abnormalities on a CAT scan that were not seen on MRI was 0 percent, whereas the probability of a positive MRI when the CAT scan was unrevealing was 80 percent. An MRI is more useful than a CAT scan with contrast for the investigation of epilepsy. Gadolinium generally is not contributory.

When a patient has a normal CAT scan and the cause of the seizures remains obscure, an MRI with special attention to the temporal lobes is likely to provide additional information. High-resolution MRI has done much to eliminate the number of "cryptogenic" epilepsy cases. Magnetic resonance imaging has a sensitivity of 86 percent compared with surgical specimens for pathology.

Sandra's MRI confirmed the CAT scan findings of generalized atrophy, but it failed to reveal MTS or another etiology for epilepsy. Cerebral atrophy in a 34-year-old is unusual and could represent a neurodegenerative disease. Cerebral atrophy has also been associated with anorexia nervosa. Given Sandra's otherwise normal neurologic examination, I provisionally attributed this finding to her eating disorder.

There are two primary goals in the evaluation of a patient with seizures. The first is the treatment of the seizures. The second is the diagnosis and treatment of their etiology. In many cases, when the cause remains unknown, the focus of treatment remains the seizures. In other instances, such as when a brain tumor is discovered, treating the *cause* of the seizure becomes paramount.

7. Does Sandra need treatment for epilepsy?

I'm not sure yet.

Some clinicians define epilepsy as two or more unprovoked seizures occurring at least 24 hours apart. Although Sandra had three events, they all occurred on the same day, with full recovery in between. Her EEG was not definitive, and there were the possible provocations of mirtazapine and sleep deprivation.

One must try to clarify the goals of therapy. As in most cases, the goal of beginning an AED would be to prevent further seizures. Given the unique circumstances of the current seizures, it is difficult to make a prediction on the likelihood of recurrence. Most neurologists would not start AED therapy on the basis of a single seizure unless there was other information, such as an abnormal MRI scan or EEG, to suggest an underlying disease. Sandra's MRI revealed atrophy, but it did not suggest an etiology for epilepsy. Her EEG was equivocal.

Treatment would not be without risks. As many as 36 percent of patients report adverse effects from chronic AED therapy. I discussed these considerations with Sandra.

Rather than begin AED therapy, it seemed reasonable to stop the mirtazapine and try a period of watchful waiting. Sandra reluctantly consented to avoid driving and other dangerous activities in the meantime. If she had another seizure while off the mirtazapine, we would have a secure diagnosis of epilepsy and begin AED treatment. If she had no further spells, she could resume her normal activities after a month or so. We both agreed on the plan, and I documented our discussion in her chart.

Three weeks later Sandra called me from the waiting room in the local ER. She had been driving home from the unemployment office and crashed her car into a telephone pole. The last thing she remembered was that she was stopped at a red light. Sandra told me she had to leave the ER without being evaluated so she could pick up her daughter at day care. I encouraged her to stay and be assessed by a physician.

Two hours later I got a call from Sandra's neighbor. Sandra had taken a cab from the ER and returned home. Her neighbor was preparing to drive her to day care when Sandra had a generalized tonic-clonic seizure on the front porch. I asked the neighbor to call 911. I called the ER physician and advised him that Sandra would be returning. I asked him to consider repeating another CAT scan because of the motor vehicle accident and her fall off the porch. She would also need to be loaded with phenytoin and followed up in my office.

Clearly, Sandra and I were going to have to talk more about epilepsy and compliance. Her life has changed dramatically with the definite diagnosis of epilepsy and inability to drive. Her seizure disorder will only compound her personal and financial problems. She will be upset and may require counseling and social support.

8. Is there more than one type of convulsion?

Yes.

In order to properly classify her seizure type (see Resource B), it is important to know whether the convulsions are primary generalized or partial seizures with secondary generalization. Carbamazepine, phenytoin, and valproate are the most effective AEDs for partial seizures. Valproate is superior to carbamazepine and phenytoin for primary generalized seizures.

Sandra's confusional episodes may represent absence attacks or partial complex seizures. Another EEG may help discern her seizure type and direct us toward the most effective therapy. (I chose phenytoin for the moment because of the likelihood of partial seizures and the practical consideration that Sandra could receive a phenytoin load in the ER.)

Three types of classification are important when patients present with new-onset seizures. The first is the seizure type. Was it a convulsion? If so, what kind? Was it a myoclonic jerk, a partial complex seizure, an absence attack? The second question is the etiology. What caused the seizure—a brain tumor, genetics, drugs? The third question is whether a specific epilepsy syndrome can be identified, such as childhood absence, juvenile myoclonic epilepsy (JME), or partial seizures secondary to MTS.

The diagnosis of an epilepsy syndrome helps enormously with treatment decisions and prognosis. For example, childhood absence epilepsy responds well to ethosuximide or valproate. One can predict that the child will outgrow the syndrome.

Juvenile myoclonic epilepsy is characterized by teenage onset, staring spells, myoclonic jerks, and convulsions. This syndrome also tends to respond well to valproate, but it is rarely outgrown. Sleep deprivation exacerbates JME. Consequently, the physician should stress the importance of adequate rest and counsel the patient that AED therapy is likely to represent a long-term commitment.

Benign rolandic epilepsy presents with nocturnal convulsions and focal seizures of the face. Large central spikes appear on the EEG. These seizures disappear by age 16.

Seizures caused by MTS often are refractory to AEDs, but frequently are amenable to epilepsy surgery. When MRI identifies MTS in an intractable epilepsy patient, prompt referral to a comprehensive epilepsy center may result in dramatic improvement.

I still have much to learn about Sandra's epilepsy. The recurrence of her seizures three weeks after stopping mirtazapine and my failure to identify any other provoking factor suggest that she has true epilepsy. I don't know whether she had a convulsion or a confusional spell in her car.

It may be possible to define Sandra's epilepsy syndrome as more information becomes available. This will help with prognosis and with the next question she will ask: How long do I have to take medication for my epilepsy? (See Chapter 3.)

2

Intractable Epilepsy

Daniel's mother feared that his seizures would never go away. Her pregnancy, now 40 years ago, had passed without incident, but birth was premature by six weeks, and the baby was blue. Daniel didn't walk until 16 months, six months later than his brother. He couldn't speak sentences until he was three years old.

His first convulsion occurred in his crib when he was 15 months old. Sometimes he seemed afraid and would run to his mother. Other times he suddenly convulsed violently. The doctor treated him with phenobarbital and phenytoin for many years. He was switched to primidone at the age of 12 and became violent. He attacked a neighbor with a hatchet and was institutionalized. When the primidone was stopped, his behavior improved, and he returned home at age 18. Two years ago, while taking valproate, he again became aggressive. The medication was changed to lamotrigine, and he resumed his usual placid disposition.

Over the years he has failed acetazolamide, carbamazepine, chlordiazepoxide, clorazepate, diazepam, ethosuximide, phenobarbital, phenytoin, primidone, and valproate. He continues to have seizures approximately three times per month on a combination of phenytoin and lamotrigine. He once had status epilepticus after several days of gastroenteritis with nausea and vomiting because he could not keep down his medications.

Danny takes medications for high blood pressure and hypothyroidism. He has had numerous lacerations on his face and scalp from falls resulting from seizures. He fractured each wrist on separate occasions, and he recently broke his right foot.

He has no allergies, and does not smoke, drink, or abuse drugs. No one else in the family has epilepsy. His mother is afraid to let him try to live independently because of his seizures and his lack of cognitive and social skills. She does everything for him. At the age of 40, he has never done laundry, cooked a meal, managed a checkbook, or left the house on his own to go farther than his mother can see him. He is single and does not have any significant dating relationships. He is receiving disability benefits, and he does not drive.

As she gets older, his mother worries about what will happen to her son when she's gone. Her husband, Daniel's stepfather, doesn't show much interest in him.

On examination, Daniel is slow to answer but appropriate. When asked a question, his favorite answer seems to be, "I'm still kicking." Mini-Mental State Exam score is 25/30. Medical examination is remarkable for a cast on his right foot. Neurologic examination is nonfocal, without evidence of weakness, numbness, speech difficulty, or visual field defect to point to a specific brain lesion.

Questions

9. Does Daniel have intractable epilepsy?

Yes.

A single antiepileptic drug (AED) controls seizures in 70 percent of patients with epilepsy. Another 15 percent achieve control with two or three medications. Few patients benefit from three or more concurrent AEDs. If monotherapy trials do not control seizures within two years, success with monotherapy is unlikely. Daniel has tried various combinations of seven AEDs, as well as three benzodiazepines.

Daniel's seizures are characterized by convulsions and feelings of fear. He most likely has partial seizures that can secondarily generalize into generalized tonic-clonic convulsions. His seizure type suggests temporal lobe epilepsy. Consequently, he has a localization-related epilepsy syndrome, possibly related to a difficult birth. Further investigation may clarify the syndrome and help direct treatment and prognosis.

A better understanding of epilepsy, new AEDs, refined surgical techniques, and alternative therapies all would justify an accelerated treatment plan to control seizures as soon as possible, compared with Daniel's prior management. There are many reasons for this:

- Intractable epilepsy may be responsible for progressive cognitive impairment.

- Detrimental social consequences of recurrent seizures increase with time and can become irreversible.
- Seizures may become more difficult to control with time.
- Functional recovery is likely to be greater when brain surgery is performed at a younger age.
- A high seizure frequency is an important risk factor for sudden unexplained death in epilepsy.

A suggested treatment timeline appears below:

Timeline for Seizure Treatment

0–3 months—Monotherapy AED trials with first-line medications (carbamazepine, phenytoin, valproate)

3 months—Neurologist referral; begin trials with newer AEDs (gabapentin, lamotrigine, levetiracetam, oxcarbazepine, tiagabine, and topiramate)

12 months—Referral to epilepsy center for comprehensive evaluation of epilepsy etiology, seizure type, epilepsy syndrome, neuropsychological and social services assessment

12–24 months—Consider epilepsy surgery

24 months—If patient is not a surgical candidate, consider investigative drug trials, vagal nerve stimulator, or ketogenic diet (especially for children)

10. Why are Daniel's seizures so difficult to control?

We need to know the etiology of his seizures to answer this question.

Patients with persistent seizures may not respond to AEDs for a number of reasons. In some cases, patients have been misdiagnosed and actually have another disease, such as breath-holding spells, migraine, syncope, or a movement disorder. Approximately 20 percent of patients referred to epilepsy centers have nonepileptic seizures related to psychiatric problems (see Chapter 11). Some patients have true epilepsy but have received the wrong drugs because of a misdiagnosis of seizure type. For example, carbamazepine can worsen absence seizures, whereas ethosuximide or valproate usually control them quite easily. Lack of diagnosis of the appropriate epilepsy syndrome, such as juvenile myoclonic epilepsy, also leads to errors in treatment and prognosis.

Misdiagnosis seems unlikely in Daniel's case. He has tried enough medications over the years to address both primary generalized and partial seizures. His mother is so attentive to his care that medication noncompliance has not been a problem.

Risk factors for intractable epilepsy include arteriovenous malformations, cerebral malformations, brain tumors, encephalitis, meningitis, mental retardation, severe head injury, tuberous sclerosis, and Sturge-Weber syndrome. Daniel was hypoxic at birth and had developmental delay, but we do not know the cause of his seizures. Neurologic examination reveals mild global cognitive deficits, but seizures appear to have a focal onset. He needs further work-up to clarify why his seizures are so difficult to control.

11. Will finding an etiology help Daniel after all these years of seizures?

Yes.

Daniel needs at least an electroencephalogram (EEG) and a high-resolution magnetic resonance imaging (MRI) scan. The EEG may confirm the epilepsy syndrome. It also may reveal subclinical seizures that could be interfering with Daniel's daily activities. If multiple bursts of generalized spike wave appear, rather than the suspected focal abnormalities, AED treatment will differ, and the proposed underlying etiology of temporal lobe epilepsy must be reconsidered.

Daniel's EEG was normal, which suggests that he does not have a severe encephalopathy. A large part of his disturbed cognitive and psychosocial functioning may be due to a combination of seizures, medication effects, and environmental conditions.

The MRI revealed unequivocal mesial temporal sclerosis (MTS) on the right side. One could see atrophy of the right hippocampus, with increased signal on the T2-weighted image. The ipsilateral temporal horn also was increased in size. Many patients with MTS have seizures that are difficult to control. The cause of MTS is not clear.

Because of the MRI findings, Daniel was admitted to the hospital for long-term video-EEG monitoring. We recorded eight seizures on scalp EEG. He grimaced and began chewing at the beginning of each seizure. These movements produced extensive muscle artifact, which obscured the electrographic onset of his seizures.

Daniel had a positron emission tomography (PET) scan to see whether it confirmed interictal hypometabolism in the right temporal lobe. The scan was normal.

He was readmitted to the hospital for depth electrode placement. A neurosurgeon inserted these electrodes precisely using a stereotactic frame and coordinates obtained from a computerized axial tomography (CAT) scan. Two electrodes, each with six contacts, recorded from the frontal lobes. Two more electrodes, each with eight recording contacts, sampled the temporal lobes.

During the next two weeks, while taking reduced doses of AEDs, 13 of Daniel's typical seizures were recorded on video-EEG. After studying the tracings, I determined that 12 of them originated in his right temporal lobe. I wasn't sure about the last one.

Extensive neuropsychological testing did not lateralize or localize an area of brain dysfunction. (A specific neuropsychological abnormality such as poor verbal versus visuospatial abilities often coincides with the seizure focus.) Daniel had an IQ of 83. He had a Wada (sodium amytal) test to determine his dominant hemisphere and evaluate short-term memory of each temporal lobe. The test indicated that he was left language-dominant. Using his left hemisphere, Daniel remembered 11 of 12 items. Using his right hemisphere, he didn't get any answers correct.

The MRI, depth electrode seizure recordings, and Wada test results all pointed to the right temporal lobe as the seizure focus. The MRI was not sufficient evidence on which to base a surgical resection because some patients have bilateral MTS or additional seizure foci.

The risks and benefits of a temporal lobectomy were explained to Daniel and his parents. Postoperative hemorrhage, cerebral infarct, and wound infections occur infrequently. Because Daniel's speech center was in the left temporal lobe, opposite his seizure focus, a right temporal lobectomy would not threaten his language ability. A temporal lobectomy *would* interfere with the optic pathway fibers of Meyer's loop and predictably cause a superior quadrantanopia in the left visual field. The anesthesiologist did not think that Daniel's hypertension and hypothyroidism represented significant operative risks.

Epilepsy surgery is reserved for patients who have failed medical treatment and whose seizures significantly interfere with their lives. With much reluctance, Daniel's mother agreed. She could see that he had more to gain than to lose from the operation.

Daniel said he would do anything to get rid of his seizures because he wanted to be "normal" and stop taking medication. The neuropsychologist cautioned him that even if the surgery were a success, it would still take some work before he could get a job and move out of the house. It also was likely that he would stay on at least one AED for some time.

Daniel's last seizure occurred during his depth electrode monitoring. He has been seizure-free since his surgery six years ago.

12. Are there other types of epilepsy surgery

Yes.

Anterior temporal lobectomy is the most commonly performed epilepsy surgery. Extratemporal surgery, in the frontal, parietal, or occipital lobes, can also improve seizure frequency but has a lower overall success rate. The success of resective epilepsy surgery depends on accurate preoperative identification of the seizure focus. Localization can be fairly certain if there is a lesion on imaging studies, such as MTS, as in Daniel's case, or, for example, a brain tumor in the frontal lobe that agrees with EEG findings. If there is no visible lesion, more reliance shifts to the EEG recordings; functional imaging studies, such as PET and single photon emission computed tomography (SPECT); and neuropsychological testing for accurate lateralization and localization.

Patients who have multiple seizure foci are not good candidates for resective epilepsy surgery. Lesions in "eloquent" brain areas, such as Wernicke's speech area in the temporal lobe or the motor strip in the frontal lobe, present special challenges. Surgery in these regions requires meticulous functional brain mapping and may be perilous.

Some children have such a badly damaged hemisphere that its removal or disconnection can improve seizures and developmental outcome. Because the affected hemisphere is already severely impaired, resulting in hemianopsia, hemiparesis, and other dysfunction, surgical removal of the hemisphere may not result in additional deficits. This operation, a hemispherectomy, was first performed for seizures in 1938. When the hemisphere is left in place but disconnected, the procedure is called a functional hemispherectomy. Candidates for this type of surgery usually are children with intractable epilepsy due to cerebral infarcts, hemimegalencephaly, infantile hemiplegic epilepsy, Rasmussen's encephalitis, or Sturge-Weber syndrome.

Early hemispherectomy may improve psychosocial functioning. A multilobar resection rather than a hemispherectomy may be sufficient for some patients.

Another type of epilepsy surgery is corpus callosotomy. The primary indication for this procedure is intractable drop attacks. This operation can also help patients who have secondarily generalized seizures. Disconnection of the major white matter tracts between the two hemispheres hinders the rapid generalization of electrical discharges and prevents the patient from falling abruptly. Sectioning the corpus callosum also may decrease convulsions in children who have multiple epileptic foci and frequent secondarily generalized convulsions. Corpus callosotomy is a palliative procedure that is employed when resection of an epileptic focus is not an option.

To avoid a "split-brain" syndrome, the neurosurgeon usually sections only the anterior portion of the corpus callosum. (If necessary, the operation can be completed at a later time by sectioning the splenium.) Corpus callosotomy rarely renders patients seizure-free. However, the elimination or reduction of drop attacks or convulsions may decrease injuries and greatly improve quality of life. Significant neuropsychological deficits from the surgery are uncommon.

13. Was Daniel "normal" after his temporal lobectomy?

No.

Before the surgery, the neuropsychologist noted that Daniel had failed to develop socially in many ways, in large part because his mother was overprotective. Although he was not mentally retarded, his IQ was significantly below average. He had received little formal schooling because he was institutionalized during his high school years. Daniel failed to achieve the normal developmental accomplishments of adolescence, such as a sense of physical, academic, or social competence. He has socialized with his peers only in a very limited way. Daily medication for as long as he can remember has served as a constant reminder of his illness, and he suffers from low self-esteem.

Social problems, particularly anxiety, poor self-concept, social isolation, and depression, are common in people with epilepsy. In many ways he still suffers from the illness of epilepsy, even without his seizures.

Daniel has learned to drive a car since his surgery. He now has increased mobility and can visit friends and run errands. He has no work skills that might lead to employment. He experiences frustration when he tries to learn things and realizes that even without seizures, his abilities are limited. Although MTS was the only lesion visible on his MRI scan, he appears to have a mild static encephalopathy as well.

Recognizing the limitations imposed by epilepsy, many parents restrict the activities and peer interactions of their children. Although this is understandable, the psychosocial consequences of this behavior may be as severe as the seizures. I have interviewed many patients in their twenties and thirties who acted like children in the examining room. This developmental arrest is partially due to limited abilities, but it may be unnecessarily exaggerated by well-meaning parents.

The goal of treatment for all patients is to enable them to function at their full potential. Elimination of the seizures is but one part of the treatment for patients with chronic epilepsy. Early intervention with medication or surgical therapy can eliminate seizures before chronic social dysfunction becomes an irreversible way of life. In addition, there is mounting evidence that repeated seizures result in increased brain injury. Interictal behavioral disturbances (see Chapter 7) may be less likely to appear if the seizures are stopped promptly.

Many patients like Daniel express unrealistic expectations of epilepsy surgery. It is critical to make certain that both the patient and the family understand the intended goals of the operation. Most patients require at least one AED as adjunctive therapy, even after successful temporal lobectomy. Reversing the social limitations of lifelong epilepsy is a much more difficult task than performing a temporal lobectomy.

14. Is there anything that can help Daniel adapt to his new life?

Yes.

A surgical success may be as psychologically traumatic to a patient as a surgical failure. I have seen one patient develop pseudoseizures postoperatively (see Chapter 11), because she was so overwhelmed by living without epilepsy for the first time. Other patients divorce because of dramatic changes in their relationship dynamics. To a large extent, these reactions can be anticipated.

I insist that all patients see a neuropsychologist before temporal lobectomy, not only for testing, but also for counseling. Patients should also have postoperative sessions with the neuropsychologist to allow them to discuss feelings about the surgical outcome, whether positive or negative. Patients are sometimes reluctant to express disappointment or recount difficulties to their neurologist or neurosurgeon, but they will talk more openly with a neuropsychologist. The neuropsychologist can better assess postoperative problems when a therapeutic relationship has been established with the patient preoperatively. Patients also often benefit from the input of a psychiatrist and a social worker.

Many patients profit from speaking to peers who have had epilepsy surgery. Epilepsy support groups exist throughout the country and help patients put their prospective surgery in perspective. Brain surgery can be a daunting proposition. It can be comforting to learn that others have experienced and benefited from it. In a support group, patients have an opportunity to voice concerns about surgery, relationships, and opinions about caregivers, as well as to address practical needs such as transportation and obtaining low-cost medication, in a protected environment. The Epilepsy Foundation has many chapters throughout the country that provide information on jobs for patients with epilepsy, local support groups, and transportation services (see Resource AB). Other local and international resources (see Resource AC) are also available.

Daniel could probably have benefited from a sheltered workshop before his operation. Training Applicants for Placement Success (TAPS), a nationwide job program for patients with epilepsy that is funded by the U.S. Department of Labor, might be able to place him in a manageable work environment. He has been to vocational rehabilitation but has not yet found a job. Unemployment is increased at least two to three times for people with epilepsy. Intractable seizures are only partially responsible for this problem; limited education and skills, associated neurologic and psychological deficits, lack of access to transportation, and employer attitudes contribute to underemployment.

Daniel continues to live at home since his surgery. He attended adult education classes and passed his high school equivalency test after three years. He has volunteered at the local hospital for the last two years.

Daniel has made a few friends in the local epilepsy support group. It is difficult for his mother to let him leave the house without her, but she is no longer afraid that he will injure himself as a result of a seizure. His stepfather took him fishing for the first time.

15. Were there other options for Daniel besides surgery?

Yes. The first is additional medication trials with approved or investigational drugs.

Temporal lobectomy can achieve dramatic results in patients with epilepsy. The key to success is careful patient selection by an experienced epileptologist, neurosurgeon, and epilepsy team. At most comprehensive epilepsy centers, patients are presented in a multidisciplinary conference for discussion before surgery. Patients who do the best have a single seizure focus, a definite MRI scan abnormality, EEG recordings that localize to the same area, and relatively high psychosocial functioning. Those who do the worst have more than one seizure focus, either no apparent lesion on MRI or more than one, EEGs with unclear findings or multiple seizure foci, and low psychosocial functioning. Like many patients, Daniel falls somewhere in between.

The new age of AEDs has enormously increased the number of possible medication options. It would take a lifetime to try every possible AED combination. Consequently, it is important not to waste too much time experimenting with each marketed drug. For partial onset seizures, trials of at least two of the newer drugs (gabapentin, lamotrigine, levetiracetam, oxcarbazepine, tiagabine, and topiramate) should be performed before considering surgery.

Another consideration is investigational medication. Before an AED can be licensed by the U.S. Food and Drug Administration (FDA), it must be tested in Phase III trials on a large number of patients to demonstrate safety and efficacy. Trained investigators perform these trials under strict protocols. Patients usually receive investigational medication at no charge and also are provided free study-related health care. This usually includes frequent physician visits, serum chemistries, blood count, urinalysis, and AED levels. Patients benefit from the close attention they receive during a clinical trial. A placebo response often occurs, resulting in fewer seizures. Unfortunately, experience has shown that only a few patients become seizure-free on protocol medication when they have failed multiple other drugs.

16. Is the vagal nerve stimulator effective?

Yes.

The first vagal nerve stimulator (VNS) implant was performed in 1988. After nine years of testing, the FDA approved the VNS in 1997. Extensive clinical experience has been obtained with this "neurocybernetic prosthesis." As of July 1997, more than 1,000 patients have been implanted. In the operating room, a neurosurgeon wraps a delicate electrode around the left vagus nerve and connects it to a programmable pacemaker-like device inserted in a subcutaneous pocket in the chest. The procedure can be done on an outpatient basis, but inpatient observation after the procedure is prudent because of the proximity of the vagus nerve to the carotid artery.

The exact mechanism behind the efficacy of the vagal stimulator is not known. Afferent fibers of the vagus nerve project to the solitary tract, reticular formation, dorsal motor nucleus of the vagus, area postrema, and the cuneate nucleus. The ambiguous nucleus, amygdala, dorsal raphe, hypothalamus, parabrachial nucleus, and thalamus all receive inputs from the solitary tract nucleus. Consequently, the VNS can have widespread influence in many brain structures. It affects autonomic reflexes, cortical excitability, electroencephalographic synchronization, and sleep cycles. Gamma-aminobutyric acid (GABA) and glycine may be released in the brainstem and cerebral cortex as a result of VNS. Vagal nerve stimulation decreases interictal spike frequency and seizure duration in rats.

The neurologist programs the VNS with a laptop computer to provide pulses of intermittent stimulation of the vagus nerve 24 hours a day. For example, it may stimulate for 30 seconds "on," then 5 minutes "off." The programmer can adjust the amplitude, frequency, and current duration to patient tolerance. In addition, a patient can wave an external magnet over the device to trigger a discharge during an aura. This may abort a seizure.

Efficacy varies among patients. Overall, seizures decrease approximately 30 percent with the VNS, which is similar to the effect of newer AEDs. Approximately one third of all patients have a greater than 50 percent seizure reduction. Unlike many AEDs, however, the VNS does not have cognitive or teratogenic side effects. The VNS is not adversely affected by airport security systems, cellular phones, or microwaves. Because of the possibility of heat generation due to a conventional MRI study, these scans are contraindicated once VNS electrodes have been surgically implanted.

Patients may cough or become hoarse when the VNS triggers. Surgical problems are extremely rare but may include wound infection and injury to the recurrent laryngeal nerve. At standard stimulation settings, the lithium battery lasts longer than six years. Patients rarely become seizure-free.

17. Is the ketogenic diet worth trying?

In children, definitely yes. In adults, maybe.

The ketogenic diet was pioneered more than 75 years ago. When phenytoin and ethosuximide became available, enthusiasm for the diet waned in favor of these more facile solutions for seizure control. In the past few years, however, the ketogenic diet has received renewed attention for the treatment of intractable epilepsy by patients, their families, and neurologists. Clinical trials have confirmed its efficacy in selected patients. (Because the diet is now so well accepted among epileptologists, I did not include it as an "alternative therapy" in Chapter 12.)

The ketogenic diet is rich in fat and very low in carbohydrate and protein. The nature of the diet forces the body to burn fat rather than glucose. It is believed that acidosis, dehydration, and the effect of ketones on the brain contribute to seizure control, but no definite mechanism of action has been identified.

The diet must be individualized. A specially trained dietitian initiates the diet during a brief inpatient hospital stay. To prepare for the diet, patients fast to become ketotic. Blood glucose is monitored to detect hypoglycemia. To sustain ketosis, the diet is usually a 4:1 ratio of fat to carbohydrate and protein (4 grams of fat plus 1 gram of carbohydrate and protein). This ratio must be maintained at each meal. The patient and/or parents must learn to weigh food items on a gram scale and calculate calories to prepare meals. Strict adherence to the diet is essential for success.

A typical meal is based on 75 percent of the recommended calories for a child's age and ideal body weight in kilograms. To simplify calculations and provide a varied diet, there are six basic meal plans:

1. Meat/fish/poultry, fruit, fat, cream
2. Cheese, fruit, fat, cream

3. Egg, fruit, fat, cream
4. Meat/fish/poultry, vegetables, fat, cream
5. Cheese, vegetables, fat, cream
6. Egg, vegetables, fat, cream

For example, a tuna salad lunch for a nine-year-old boy with an ideal body weight of 29 kilograms consists of 80 grams of 36 percent cream, 35 grams of group B vegetables (such as beets, broccoli, or spinach), 32 grams of tuna fish, and 24 grams of mayonnaise. The cream and mayonnaise provide a large part of the fat needed to maintain ketosis.

The diet must be strictly followed. A cookie, a piece of chocolate, or even the sweetener in a child's toothpaste may result in the loss of ketosis and breakthrough seizures.

In a Johns Hopkins series of children with mental retardation, cerebral palsy, and mixed seizure types, 29 percent of children were nearly seizure-free on the ketogenic diet, and 38 percent had better than 50 percent improvement. Ten percent of the children discontinued all AEDs.

Serum lipids increase on the diet, although the long-term effects of this are not known. Renal lithiasis occurs in approximately 5 percent of children. Acetazolamide and topiramate—carbonic anhydrase inhibitors that can induce metabolic acidosis—should be avoided during treatment with the ketogenic diet.

Not surprisingly, adults do not find the diet very palatable. The small portions can result in hunger and irritability. Constipation is not uncommon. Adults who adhere to the diet may see an improvement in their seizures. By far the most common use is in children, particularly those with multiple handicaps and intractable epilepsy.

Patients on the diet should receive multivitamins and calcium supplements. If children become seizure-free, the diet can often be discontinued after two years without seizure recurrence. Motivated patients should be referred to a comprehensive epilepsy center for a trial of the ketogenic diet. Practical information for patients considering the ketogenic diet can be found in *The Ketogenic Diet: A Treatment for Epilepsy*, 3rd edition, New York: Demos Medical Publishing, Inc., 2000.

3

Stopping Antiepileptic Medications

Jack is a 37-year-old man who has been seizure-free for 10 years and would like to stop taking his antiepileptic medication. Because of Jack's high-profile job, my partner asked for my opinion.

Jack had an uneventful gestation, birth, and development. He rode a motorcycle during adolescence and had several accidents. In one of them, he struck a telephone pole and was unconscious for an hour. He was observed in the hospital overnight and had a normal computed axial tomography (CAT) scan.

Uncertain about his career goals, Jack dropped out of college and diverted his attention to drugs and alcohol. He occasionally used intravenous cocaine and heroin. For the most part he relied on large quantities of beer and small amounts of sniffed cocaine to get through the day.

Late one Sunday morning, after celebrating his 21st birthday, his roommate heard gasping and snorting noises and found Jack thrashing on the floor trapped between the wall and his bed. Terrified, he called 911. The emergency medical technicians injected some kind of medication into Jack's vein for what they said was an epileptic convulsion. By the time they loaded him into the ambulance, the jerking movements had stopped.

In the emergency room (ER), Jack's drug screen was positive for alcohol, cocaine, and marijuana. A CAT scan was negative. When he woke up a few hours later, the ER physician told him to stop using illicit drugs and follow up with his primary care physician. Jack didn't do either.

Two months later, again on a Sunday morning, he had another convulsion. He bit his tongue and soiled his clothes. His roommate called 911 and Jack was transported back to the hospital. His neurologic examination was unremarkable. Another CAT scan was negative. This time the ER doctor loaded him with intravenous phenytoin and gave him a prescription for 300 mg per/day. Jack filled the prescription and took the orange-striped white capsules when he remembered.

Jack experienced four or five more convulsions over the next two years, usually early in the morning after a night of partying. If his roommate was home, he called 911 and the ambulance took Jack to the hospital. The ER doctor always said that the phenytoin level was low. If the seizure occurred when he was alone, Jack just lay on the floor until he woke up, usually with a bad headache.

He had a seizure while awake on only one occasion. First he noted a flashing light on the right side, and then he lost consciousness.

When he was 23 years old, Jack met a girl who inspired him to refocus his energies. After a few false starts, he stopped abusing drugs and cut down drastically on his alcohol intake. He took his phenytoin religiously. He returned to college and graduated. Jack went to business school and got a master's degree in healthcare administration. He and his girlfriend got married and had two children.

When he completed graduate school at age 27, Jack had been seizure-free for four years. He and his wife celebrated with dinner and champagne. Jack decided he didn't need phenytoin anymore and stopped taking it when the prescription ran out.

Two weeks later he startled his wife with a convulsion as he got dressed for work. A CAT scan in the ER was normal. He had an electroencephalogram that showed slow waves and a question of sharp transients. A magnetic resonance scan was normal. His family doctor instructed him to resume his phenytoin. For the last 10 years, Jack has been raising his family, working his way up the corporate ladder, taking his medication, and free of seizures.

Last year he saw my partner and complained that the medication caused his gums to bleed. He also thought it made his thinking "foggy," but he had been on it so long he wasn't sure. Over a period of a few weeks, he switched uneventfully to divalproex sodium, 750 mg/day.

Yesterday Jack was promoted to corporate vice president of my hospital network. He anticipates longer hours and more travel. The valproate costs almost three times as much as the phenytoin and he is concerned about the expense. Antiepileptic medication is not covered by his health insurance because his epilepsy was a "preexisting condition." My partner told him he was lucky his seizures were controlled on divalproex sodium because the newer epilepsy drugs cost even more.

Jack has been under a great deal of stress because of increasing expenses. His children both attend private school and he is building a waterfront summer home. He has encouraged his wife to go back to work, but she has not yet made a decision. Jack has been taking ser-traline for depression for the last six months. He has severe headaches about once a month. He has always had a tremor of his hands, but he is sure it is worse since he started the divalproex sodium. He says it makes him look like he is nervous at meetings when he isn't.

Jack has no history of febrile seizures, myoclonic jerks, encephalitis, or meningitis. He remembers that he got into a fight once in a bar and was unconscious for an hour or so, but he doesn't know whether the loss of consciousness was from a concussion or intoxication with drugs or alcohol. The only family member with a history of epilepsy is his son, who had a single febrile seizure.

His current medications are divalproex sodium, 750 mg/day, sertra-line, 100 mg/day, and a butalbital-aspirin-caffeine combination pain reliever for headaches.

Jack has no allergies, and he doesn't smoke, drink, or use drugs. He frequently drives to the airport, as well as to the five local hospitals that form our healthcare network. He visits the construction site of his summer home at least three times a week to supervise the builders.

Jack appears nervous on examination. His vital signs are unremark-able. One can see mild gingival hypertrophy when he smiles. He has a postural tremor and a slight tremor of his head. The rest of his exami-nation is normal.

Questions

18. Does Jack have epilepsy?

Yes.

Before we can even address the question of whether Jack needs antiepileptic drug (AED) treatment, we must decide whether he has epilepsy and, if so, try to determine the seizure type and syndrome. Then we need to look at the cost of continuing medications, both finan-cial and social, versus the medical and social consequences of another seizure for this particular patient.

Drugs, alcohol, and sleep deprivation were associated with all of Jack's seizures in his early twenties. Given the clear provocation for each seizure, his normal neurologic examination and CAT scans, and the lack of epileptic activity on his electroencephalogram (EEG), one could not make the diagnosis of epilepsy with certainty.

Jack's last convulsion occurred at age 27, when he stopped his phenytoin. The abrupt drop in his phenytoin level may have precipi-tated this seizure.

One interesting feature of his seizures is that all but one occurred in the early morning upon awakening, which suggests that he might have "epilepsy with grand mal seizures upon awakening," a generalized epilepsy with a strong genetic component. This syndrome has a male preponderance, with seizures often triggered by sleep deprivation or alcohol; it presents in late childhood, adolescence, or early adulthood, and is associated with irresponsible behavior. Neurologic development is normal, and generalized spike and wave appears on the EEG.

Jack had a total of approximately six convulsions upon awakening, the minimum required for a definite diagnosis. He did not begin to have seizures until his twenties, which, although later than most patients with this syndrome, is still within the reported range.

Patients whose only seizure type is a grand mal convulsion are difficult to classify. Grand mal seizures occur in primary generalized epilepsies, but also as a result of secondary generalization from a focus in localization-related epilepsies. What may be a critical feature in Jack's history is the one seizure he had with a visual aura, suggesting a focal seizure from the occipital lobe with secondary generalization. If an occipital lobe lesion causes his seizures, this changes our management and prognostic expectations.

Regardless of his epilepsy syndrome, Jack has learned that sleep deprivation, drugs, and alcohol trigger seizures. By eliminating these provoking factors and consistently taking his antiepileptic medication, he has successfully prevented seizures for the last 10 years. The challenging question now is whether he has epilepsy.

19. Would a repeat electroencephalogram be useful?

Yes. To optimize treatment and prognosis, we still need to know whether he has focal or primary generalized seizures.

Jack's first electroencephalogram (EEG) was nonspecific. It did not reveal the generalized spike and wave or photosensitivity that are characteristic of grand mal seizures upon awakening. Neither did it provide evidence for occipital lobe epilepsy, however. Slow waves can be seen in any type of epilepsy as well as in toxic and metabolic conditions. Their presence is not very helpful in differential diagnosis except to confirm an organic abnormality, suggesting that seizures are truly epileptic and not functional. A "question of sharp transients" is not definitive enough to be helpful (see Resource Z).

Additional EEGs might shed some light on the etiology of his seizures. Focal occipital spikes would point toward a localization-related epilepsy, whereas generalized spike and wave would be consistent with a primary generalized disorder.

At least 40 percent of patients with grand mal seizures upon awakening have generalized spike and wave on the EEG. Hyperventilation and photic stimulation tend to trigger spike and wave discharges in these patients. Even though Jack has been seizure-free for 10 years, a definite diagnosis of epilepsy with grand mal seizures upon awakening would cause me to recommend that he continue his antiepileptic medication because this syndrome is rarely outgrown.

Alternatively, the discovery of focal slowing, sharp waves, or spikes in the occipital lobe would suggest a focal epileptic cortical lesion. Because his magnetic resonance imaging (MRI) scan was performed with 10-year-old technology, I would order another scan to look for a lesion that might have been missed or one that has evolved in the interim. The presence of a structural lesion would also support a recommendation to continue AED treatment.

Jack needs to have a sleep-deprived EEG. If that does not provide any diagnostic information, a prolonged ambulatory EEG such as a DigiTrace could be helpful. If his MRI and EEGs are normal, his prognosis is considerably improved and we may consider a trial of gradual medication withdrawal.

20. Is head injury the cause of Jack's seizures?

Probably not.

Head injury is a major risk factor, accounting for approximately 5 percent of all cases of epilepsy. Posttraumatic epilepsy occurs more often in men than in women. Penetrating wounds caused by missiles (usually bullets) are much more likely to produce seizures than are closed head injuries. Risk factors for seizures caused by penetrating head injuries include an abnormal neurologic examination, brain volume loss, intracranial hematoma, and retained metal fragments. In general, the more severe the injury, the more likely epilepsy will develop.

Jack had at least one significant head injury from his motorcycle accident and possibly another after an altercation. He did not have prolonged amnesia (greater than 24 hours) or coma, which increase the likelihood of developing epilepsy. Intraparenchymal bleeding exposes the brain to hemosiderin and iron's epileptogenic effect. The absence of hemorrhage or depressed skull fracture on his CAT scan confirms a lack of structural injury.

Only about 5 percent of patients hospitalized for nonpenetrating head injury develop seizures. More than half of these patients have their first seizure within 12 months of the injury. Jack's seizures occurred approximately three years after his motorcycle injury and one year after his barroom brawl.

Many patients with seizure disorders mistakenly believe that a remote childhood head injury is the cause of their epilepsy. The severity and temporal relationship of the injury to seizure onset are the best indicators of a causal relationship.

21. Is divalproex sodium the right treatment for grand mal seizures upon awakening?

Yes.

Divalproex sodium (Depakote) is an excellent drug for primary generalized epilepsies. These include childhood absence epilepsy, juvenile absence epilepsy, juvenile myoclonic epilepsy, epilepsy with grand mal seizures upon awakening, and others. Generalized spike and wave on the electroencephalogram characterizes these epilepsies. Other drugs, such as the barbiturates and phenytoin, may also be effective for grand mal seizures upon awakening.

For partial seizures, such as occur from an occipital lesion, most epileptologists would recommend phenytoin or carbamazepine, with valproate as a second choice. Lamotrigine and oxcarbazepine have recently been approved for monotherapy treatment of partial seizures.

22. Jack has been seizure-free for 10 years. Isn't that long enough to wait before withdrawing antiepileptic medications?

Not if he has grand mal seizures upon awakening, a syndrome that tends to last for many years.

Because every patient is unique, generalizations about when to stop an AED are only guidelines. Most studies are confounded by heterogeneous patient samples.

Many physicians consider tapering AEDs after a patient has been seizure-free for two years. A more conservative approach is to wait four years. In one study of patients who withdrew from therapy after four seizure-free years, 24 percent had recurrent seizures. In population studies from developing countries, 50 percent of patients with seizures spontaneously remit.

Unfortunately, although they provide "ballpark" figures, these studies are insufficient to guide the management of an individual patient. The best information comes when a particular syndrome can be identified, as discussed previously. If the patient's symptoms do not fit a clearly defined syndrome, one must rely on a number of prognostic indicators.

Factors that suggest seizures will not recur after a seizure-free interval:

- Normal neurologic examination
- Few seizures before control
- Long seizure-free interval on medication
- Normal EEG
- Normal imaging study

Factors that predict seizure relapse:

- Onset during adolescence
- Abnormal neurologic examination
- Learning disability
- Mental retardation
- History of infantile spasms
- Seizures caused by head trauma, stroke, or central nervous system infection
- Breakthrough seizures with fever
- Multiple drugs required to control seizures
- A large number of seizures before remission
- Multiple seizure types
- A long duration of epilepsy before control
- Prolonged seizures
- Abnormal EEG

Some of these risk factors are more helpful than others in terms of prediction. For example, onset during adolescence suggests genetic epilepsy, likely to be lifelong, or an acquired cause such as head trauma rather than a benign childhood epilepsy that will be outgrown. On the other hand, an epilepsy syndrome such as Lennox-Gastaut is unlikely to remit even though it began in childhood.

Jack has a normal neurologic examination and imaging studies but a slightly abnormal EEG. His son had a single febrile seizure, which technically would not qualify as a "family history of epilepsy." But this febrile seizure raises the question whether his son will develop epilepsy later in life. A family history of epilepsy may also be a risk factor for seizure recurrence, but this currently is unclear. If Jack's repeat EEG and MRI are normal, it would be a reasonable expectation that he will not relapse off medication.

23. Are there risks of continuing antiepileptic medication?

Yes.

It is always best medical practice to use the least amount of effective medication required to achieve the desired therapeutic result. Toxic reactions from AEDs range from rash (see Chapter 6) to aplastic anemia (see Chapter 4). The one side effect Jack complains about is tremor. He appears to have an essential tremor that is exacerbated by divalproex sodium. This probably will improve with a dose reduction.

In addition, Jack takes sertraline for depression. Both sertraline and divalproex sodium are tightly protein-bound, which raises the possibility of pharmacokinetic interactions between them. (If Jack's psychiatrist wants to use divalproex sodium to treat his depression, that is another issue altogether.)

Teratogenicity is always a consideration in women of childbearing age. None of the AEDs have been demonstrated to be safe for use during gestation (see Chapter 5). There is no clinical evidence that AEDs taken by the father are teratogenic.

Jack is concerned about his medication expense. A single AED can cost as little as $5 a month for phenobarbital to more than $200 a month for one of the newer drugs. In addition, there is the cost of physician visits, periodic serum AED levels, blood counts, and chemistries. One also must consider the effort of having to take a daily medication as well as the psychological cost of viewing oneself in a "sick" role.

24. Are there risks of a trial off medication?

Yes.

In many ways, it is much more difficult to make a decision to stop an AED than to begin one, particularly in adults. A breakthrough seizure presents many potentially serious complications for an adult. Children tend to be in supervised situations, and their risk of injury is lessened. They do not risk loss of employment or driving privileges.

When a person has an epileptic seizure, there is always the risk of bodily injury. Patients suffer lacerations, fractures, burns, and occasionally significant head injuries. Although most convulsions do not result in serious injury, a breakthrough seizure may be dangerous. Status epilepticus rarely occurs in the setting of a gradual drug taper.

If a seizure occurs at an inopportune time, patients may be struck by a moving vehicle, fall off a ladder, or drown in a bathtub. Precautions must be taken to diminish these risks of injury when a patient stops medication.

Jack has been well controlled for 10 years. As a healthcare administrator, he would be embarrassed if he had a seizure in the hospital. He does not want to lose his driving license because his job depends on his ability to supervise several hospitals. He cannot risk losing his job because he has too many expenses.

In addition, Jack takes sertraline, a selective serotonin reuptake inhibitor (SSRI). This drug causes insomnia in 16 percent of patients, which may lower Jack's seizure threshold. He may already be having difficulty sleeping because of his depression. A sleep disturbance is likely to aggravate his epilepsy (if he has it).

If Jack had a perfectly normal EEG and MRI scan, it would be reasonable to gradually taper his medication. I would lower his divalproex sodium by 125 mg every week. During this time, it would be prudent if Jack could limit his driving, avoid bathing alone, and refrain from climbing and other potentially dangerous activities. If Jack were taking a barbiturate or benzodiazepine, these drugs should be tapered over at least several months.

In the meantime, as long as his tremor is the only real complaint he has from divalproex sodium, we can slightly lower his dose to see whether his tremor improves. It would also be worthwhile to check a complete blood and platelet count and liver enzyme panel to see if he has any hematologic or hepatic medication side effects. A valproate level might be useful as a baseline.

I would also remind Jack of several steps he could take to decrease the possibility of a seizure. First, he should take his medication on a regular schedule. Second, despite the stress of his promotion, he should ensure that he gets adequate rest. Third, he should consider staying home in bed during a febrile illness because he may be at risk for a seizure at that time. Fourth, he already knows to avoid excessive alcohol and drugs. Fifth, he should follow up closely with his psychiatrist in the hopes of resolving his depression and discontinuing the SSRI.

25. If Jack stops his medication, does he need to stop driving?

It would be prudent, but not practical.

When a patient with controlled seizures discontinues antiepileptic medication, I usually recommend that they limit their driving as much as possible for the first few months. Because of the lack of public transportation where most Americans live, a driving prohibition is an extremely harsh pronouncement, and in many cases, it is unlikely to be followed. In Britain, a six-month driving-free interval is recommended after antiepileptic medications are stopped. Most patients who relapse will do so during the first year off medication. Patients should avoid driving and other high risk behavior while at risk for relapse.

Unfortunately, we still have much to learn in order to accurately predict seizure recurrence. I recently saw a patient in the hospital who had two convulsions during an episode of gastroenteritis after being seizure-free off medication for 28 years!

When faced with the topic of tapering AEDs, the physician should discuss the likelihood of relapse with the patient and often with the family as well. Each patient has a different tolerance for a breakthrough seizure. In addition, patients vary in their feelings about medication side effects and cost. Using the best predictive information, physicians and patients should decide together whether to stop AEDs. Patients must also understand that even the most reasoned prediction still only represents an educated guess.

4

Seizures and Medications

Charlotte is a 23-year-old woman whose seizures began at age 10. She remembers the bright, sunny Saturday because it was also the day of her menarche. Her mother says Charlotte stared several times for 10–20 seconds and jerked both arms up toward her head.

Gestation was complicated by spotting. Delivery was at term by caesarean section because of fetal size. Birth weight was 9.9 pounds. Development was normal.

Charlotte denies olfactory, auditory, visual, abdominal, or other aura. Her seizures precede or immediately follow her menstrual period. She has never had a convulsion.

Charlotte took phenobarbital for the first year after seizures began. When she experienced no improvement, she switched to phenytoin. She began at 300 mg a day, but her seizures continued. Her doctor said that her level was low and increased the dose to 400 mg a day. Her level was still low a week later, and he prescribed five capsules a day. Although the level increased, two weeks later it was only 8 µg/ml and seizures continued. Charlotte told him that the medication bothered her gums. They gave up on the phenytoin and the doctor prescribed ethosuximide. The seizures disappeared for a few months, but then recurred.

Charlotte's doctor sent her to a specialist who diagnosed "classic catamenial epilepsy" because seizures occurred only with her periods. He recommended high doses of acetazolamide during the 10 days a month she seemed vulnerable to seizures. Charlotte thinks she had fewer seizures with this treatment, but the drug nauseated her and she stopped taking it.

Charlotte started divalproex sodium when she was 17 years old. She went five years without seizures, but they returned a few months ago. Even though the seizures were controlled, she hated the medication because her hands shook and the doctor made her get blood tests every six months to make certain she didn't develop any liver problems. To make matters worse, she gained 63 pounds. She tried dieting and lost 20 pounds, but gained it back. At her last checkup a few weeks ago, the doctor said her bleeding time was prolonged. Because of the side effects and recurrent seizures, she and her doctor decided to try something new.

She began a trial of gabapentin, but there has been no improvement in her seizures. She used to be able to predict her seizures because they were linked to her periods, but for the last few years her periods have become irregular. Mostly she has spells in the morning when she drinks coffee with her parents and only on very rare exceptions has them in the evening. She has never had one while driving. She says she sometimes has trouble concentrating during the day, but thinks that is because of the medication. She came to me because she wants to find an antiepileptic drug that will control her seizures without side effects.

Her past medical history is remarkable for anemia, leukopenia, low blood sugar, and a hernia repair. She now takes gabapentin 2100 mg/day and an iron supplement. She is allergic to sulfa and peanuts, doesn't smoke or abuse drugs, and rarely drinks. Charlotte was always a good student and attends college part-time. She is studying to be a social worker. She is single but engaged, and she is anxious to start a family.

Her physical and neurologic examinations were normal apart from her weight of 232 pounds. An electroencephalogram (EEG) performed 10 years ago showed 3–5 cycle per second spike and wave. Another EEG recorded while she was on the divalproex sodium was normal. I ordered a routine EEG and found a 5-second burst of 4 cycle per second generalized spike and wave, a subclinical seizure. Shorter bursts of spike and wave also occurred. Her computed axial tomography and magnetic resonance imaging scans were normal.

Based on the childhood onset, absence-like seizures, normal neurologic examination and imaging, and generalized epileptic activity on the EEG, it appears that Charlotte has a primary generalized epilepsy, probably childhood absence epilepsy or juvenile absence epilepsy. If gabapentin proves ineffective, it would be reasonable to try lamotrigine or topiramate.

Questions

26. **Charlotte took 200 mg of phenytoin in the morning and 300 mg in the evening, but her plasma level was only 8 µg/ml. Yet she insisted that she was compliant. Was she?**

Charlotte is very responsible. She probably was.

A number of patients dutifully swallow their prescribed 500 mg or 600 mg of phenytoin per day, yet surprisingly have levels of 10 µg/ml or less. Although noncompliance often accounts for low plasma antiepileptic drug (AED) levels, the relationship between phenytoin dose and plasma levels varies greatly among patients. In my experience, young adults and obese patients tend to have lower levels than expected.

Some patients have low levels because of poor oral absorption. Antacids and nasogastric feedings interfere with phenytoin absorption and can be responsible for low levels. Pregnant patients absorb phenytoin poorly. The phenytoin dose should be increased until one achieves the desired level. However, dose adjustments must be made cautiously, particularly as the plasma level increases.

Because of phenytoin's nonlinear pharmacokinetics, a small dose increase may result in a much higher level than expected. When a patient's plasma level is less than 10 µg/ml, it generally is safe to increase the dose by 100 mg increments. However, smaller changes using the 30 mg or 50 mg tablets should be made when the level exceeds 10 µg/ml. I prefer the 30 mg capsules because they are sustained release, like the 100 mg capsules. The 50 mg chewable tablets are not sustained release.

One common mistake in phenytoin regulation is premature measurement of plasma levels. It may take as long as four weeks for phenytoin to achieve a new steady state following a dose adjustment. Measuring the level sooner provides misleading information.

27. **Charlotte took phenytoin twice a day. Couldn't she have taken it once a day?**

Some people can, but not Charlotte.

Most patients take oral phenytoin in the form of Dilantin Kapseals, a sustained-release preparation. Consequently, if their seizure disorders are well controlled, they may succeed with once-a-day dosing. The medication is best tolerated when it is taken at bedtime.

Some patients experience toxic symptoms when plasma levels peak. Spreading the dose out during the day minimizes the peaks and concomitant side effects.

Charlotte required more than once-a-day dosing because her seizures were poorly controlled and she needed fairly constant levels. Two or three evenly spaced doses provide a more stable plasma level.

In addition, Charlotte was 11 years old when she started phenytoin. Children metabolize phenytoin more quickly than adults do. Once-a-day dosing generally is not adequate for this age group.

28. Is it safe to assume that Charlotte's difficulty concentrating is medication related?

No.

Although antiepileptic drugs (AEDs) often cause dizziness or cognitive impairment, they are not always the culprits. Clinical seizures, subclinical seizures, postictal states, metabolic disorders, other medications, or underlying brain lesions may also be responsible. To differentiate these conditions, begin with a neurologic examination to look for signs suggestive of medication toxicity, such as nystagmus or ataxia. One way to quickly reveal evidence of imbalance and poor coordination is to ask the patient to climb off the examining table and walk a few steps.

Plasma levels also help determine whether AEDs are responsible for toxic symptoms, particularly if a baseline value is available when the patient was asymptomatic. Free plasma AED levels may be necessary to obtain an accurate picture for patients who take multiple medications, have hepatic or renal insufficiency, or are pregnant (see question #38).

Patients vary dramatically in their susceptibility to the cognitive side effects of AEDs. One of my patients could not tolerate a daily dose of 400 mg of carbamazepine. (I reluctantly lowered the dose to 200 mg until the side effects disappeared.) Another patient required more than 200 mg of phenobarbital a day for seizure control, yet she and her husband assured me that she could think as clearly as ever.

An EEG may detect subtle nonconvulsive seizures, particularly in a patient with a history of frequent seizures. Charlotte's EEG revealed a single subclinical seizure as well as briefer epileptic discharges. Five seconds of spike and wave activity is long enough to impair thinking and driving.

Memory may also be affected by bursts of generalized epileptic activity. A worried woman in her twenties who believed she had outgrown her childhood seizures came to my partner's dementia clinic complaining of memory loss. An ambulatory EEG revealed frequent subclinical seizures. Her brain was otherwise normal.

Charlotte should not be working with dangerous machinery, at heights, bathing alone, or driving until her seizures are controlled. Although she thinks she only has seizures in the morning and evening, she is not aware of all of them. An ambulatory EEG study could clarify her seizure frequency. This test would be particularly valuable before allowing her to resume driving.

29. Does Charlotte have polycystic ovary syndrome?

It seems likely.

Menstrual irregularities are common in healthy women, but they are even more common in patients with epilepsy. Herzog reported that 60 percent of women with temporal lobe epilepsy had some kind of menstrual dysfunction. These women were untreated with antiepileptic drugs (AEDs).

Valproate has been associated with an increased incidence of polycystic ovary syndrome (PCOS) (see "Glossary of Terms"). Women with epilepsy who do not take valproate have also developed PCOS. Its relationship to AEDs remains unclear.

Among other problems, patients with PCOS have chronic anovulation, which would prevent Charlotte from conceiving. Charlotte should see a gynecologist for an examination and ultrasound to see whether her irregular periods and obesity are symptoms of PCOS. Because of anovulatory cycles and continuous estrogen production, PCOS may also increase seizure frequency.

Weight gain occurs in as many as 50 percent of patients on valproate, which in some cases is quite significant and distressing. Gabapentin also has been associated with weight gain, but to a lesser degree. Now that Charlotte no longer takes divalproex sodium, she may have more success with dieting.

30. What should Charlotte do when she realizes she has missed a dose of medication?

Take it.

Patients may not remember that they missed a dose until it is time for the next one. A double dose of medication may result in toxic side effects. In this situation, it is best for the patient to take the scheduled dose, then take the missed dose a few hours later.

In general, the best approach to a missed dose of medication is to make it up. Otherwise, the plasma level of the drug will remain low until repeated doses restore the steady state.

31. Why hasn't monotherapy controlled Charlotte's seizures?

I'm not sure.

Charlotte appears to have primary generalized epilepsy, which usually responds to ethosuximide or valproate. In fact, she had a great response to valproate for five years, but breakthrough seizures, tremor, and weight gain caused her to abandon the drug. The seizures may have been due to low levels as she became discouraged with side effects and less compliant.

The upward jerking of her hands suggests a myoclonic component to her absence seizures. Consequently, Charlotte may not have typical absence epilepsy but rather a related seizure type that is less responsive to medication. Valproate would still seem to be the best drug for her, but it is unlikely that she will try it again in the near future. If lamotrigine or topiramate fail to control her seizures, perhaps a drug combination will be more successful.

Monotherapy may fail for a number of reasons:

- Wrong drug for the seizure type
- Suboptimal levels
- Doses spaced too far apart
- Drug-resistant epilepsy
- Progressive neurologic disease
- Noncompliance

Monotherapy has the advantages of lower cost, simplicity, fewer side effects, and the absence of drug interactions compared with polytherapy. However, monotherapy is not effective in all patients (see Chapter 2).

32. How often should I order routine blood tests?

Only when needed.

All patients require routine screening studies before being placed on an AED to identify any underlying abnormalities and to serve as a baseline for future reference. These studies include a complete blood count with differential and platelet count, albumin, alkaline phosphatase, alanine aminotransferase, aspartate aminotransferase, bilirubin, blood urea nitrogen, calcium, creatinine, electrolytes, globulin, glucose, magnesium, phosphorus, prothrombin time, partial thromboplastin time, total protein, and uric acid.

There is a wide variety of opinion regarding the necessary frequency of routine blood monitoring once a patient has begun an AED. Although the consequences of hepatic failure and agranulocytosis are severe, their low frequency makes screening problematic. In addition, routine checks of liver enzymes and white blood cell counts do not adequately forewarn of these rare complications.

A key consideration regarding the need for laboratory monitoring is the age of the patient. Although valproic acid has been identified as etiologic in hepatic failure, a review of these cases revealed that the likelihood of this complication was greatest in patients younger than two years old, receiving polytherapy, and with neurologic abnormalities. In this population, the risk of fatal hepatic failure is 1/500. However, in normal children over the age of 10 years, the risk was near zero. The risk continues to decline with age. The overall risk is less than 1:100,000.

Monitoring liver function tests will be fruitless for most adults on valproate. On the other hand, one could make a reasonable argument supporting frequent monitoring of liver function tests in high-risk infants or adults with liver disease.

Although as many as 15 percent of patients treated with carbamazepine develop elevated liver enzymes, only 20 patients with significant hepatic complications were reported between 1978 and 1989. Testing reveals benign leukopenia in as many as 12 percent of patients on carbamazepine, yet life-threatening agranulocytosis or aplastic anemia occurs in only 1:25,000 patients. Routine checks of liver function tests and white blood cell counts do not prevent these severe idiosyncratic reactions.

Patients should be followed up symptomatically. Vomiting heralded fatal hepatic failure due to valproate more commonly than any other symptom. Clinical symptoms should be evaluated medically and with appropriate laboratory tests. Patients with known hepatic dysfunction should receive closer scrutiny. When patients are asymptomatic, I find it reassuring to repeat baseline laboratories as part of a yearly reevaluation.

33. How often should I adjust antiepileptic drugs?

It depends on the clinical circumstances.

One should reassess prescribed medication at every office visit. Between visits, review the patient's AED regimen if there is new information such as a seizure or side effect. Here is a list of questions to ask at every evaluation:

- Does the patient need more of the AED?
- Does the patient need less of the AED?
- Does the patient need a different AED?
- Has a new medication been added (by yourself or another physician) that results in a drug-drug interaction?

- Is the patient taking any nonprescription medication or supplement that interferes with AED absorption or kinetics?
- Does the patient need to have a drug level determination?
- Can the dosing regimen be simplified to improve compliance?
- Can the patient be switched to an extended-release preparation?
- Does the patient have any acute AED side effects (dizziness, ataxia)?
- Does the patient have any chronic AED side effects (weight gain, gingival hyperplasia)?
- Is the patient taking the right drug for the seizure type?
- Can the patient be switched from two AEDs to one?
- Does the patient still need an AED? (See Chapter 3.)
- Does the patient need help with compliance (counseling, pillbox, calendar, financial aid)? (See Resource V.)
- Does the patient need a prescription refill?
- Would the patient benefit from pharmaceutical samples?

34. How often should I order antiepileptic drug levels?

Levels should answer a specific question.

An emergency room physician often tells me that one of my patients had a seizure despite the fact that the AED level was within the therapeutic range. I respond that if the AED were truly therapeutic, my patient would not have had a seizure.

Drug levels guide treatment. When patients have a therapeutic level and continue to have seizures, I often increase the dose to patient tolerance. On the other hand, if seizures occur when a patient already has a level above the therapeutic range, it may be time to switch to another medication. Newer AEDs such as gabapentin, lamotrigine, levetiracetam, oxcarbazepine, tiagabine, and topiramate do not have well-established therapeutic ranges, and consequently determination of dosage must rely primarily on clinical response and toxicity.

Antiepileptic drug levels also help assess compliance. If a patient claims to take 500 mg of phenytoin a day, but the level is undetectable, compliance is a problem. If the level is only 6 µg/ml, poor absorption, rapid metabolism, or other pharmacologic variables may be responsible (see preceding).

When a new AED has been added to the regimen, it often is worthwhile to measure the level after it has attained steady state. I usually check the level of the first AED as well, because the second drug may interact with and change the level of the first.

An AED level can be very helpful in sorting out complaints of dizziness or imbalance, which may be related to drug toxicity. Many patients immediately assume that the AED is responsible, which is often—although not always—the case. A very low plasma level argues against drug toxicity as the cause of these symptoms.

It is helpful to monitor drug levels during pregnancy, at least every trimester. Drug metabolism accelerates as a woman's body changes and the fetus grows. In addition, it is important to keep the level as low as possible to limit teratogenic effects (see Chapter 5). Free levels provide better information during pregnancy (see question #38).

Antiepileptic drug levels are often necessary in the acutely ill patient. Multiple medications, varying degrees of hepatic and renal insufficiency, altered hemodynamics, and procedures such as dialysis or plasmapheresis make it impossible to accurately estimate plasma AED levels. Daily AED levels represent a more pragmatic approach.

In summary, reasons to check an AED level are:

- Continued seizures
- Compliance questions
- Toxic symptoms
- Addition of another AED
- Addition of a medication that interferes with AED metabolism (i.e., cimetidine or erythromycin) (see Resource K)
- Pregnancy
- Rapidly changing clinical situation

An isolated drug level without clinical context raises more questions than it answers. What does a phenytoin level of 22 µg/ml—called to me after hours as a "panic level" from the laboratory—mean? Does it indicate that the patient has failed phenytoin and needs to be switched to another AED? Perhaps this high level confirms my partner's suspicion of drug toxicity related to a recent dose increase? Or, was the level drawn too close to the phenytoin load that the patient received at the hospital? Perhaps the patient failed phenytoin at a lower level, but has been seizure-free without toxic symptoms at this level. Maybe the patient is not even supposed to take phenytoin, and the level is high because the patient is taking the wrong pills?

Without clinical context, a drug level is only an expensive number that fails to benefit the patient.

35. My patient took a phenytoin overdose and his level is 43 µg/ml. Can I calculate a dose adjustment to get him back into the therapeutic range?

There isn't a formula.

Although phenytoin is often listed as having a half-life of 24 hours, it increases to almost 100 hours at toxic levels. The best strategy in this circumstance is to measure the level daily and restart the drug when the level returns to the desired concentration.

If the level falls too low, there is a reliable formula for "topping off" with a partial loading dose and returning the level to the desired range (see Resource J).

36. A few weeks after I started a patient on Tegretol, his level dropped. The man is an attorney and insists he is compliant. Is he?

Yes.

Carbamazepine induces its own metabolism, a phenomenon called autoinduction. The half-life drops from 24–36 hours to 12–15 hours after treatment has begun. This process stabilizes after approximately four to six weeks. A level rechecked at this time provides a more reliable baseline for future reference.

The addition of another enzyme-inducing AED such as phenytoin can further lower the carbamazepine half-life to as little as six hours. When the half-life is this brief, multiple daily dosing can prevent excessive peaks and troughs.

37. When can I substitute a generic antiepileptic drug?

Not very often in difficult-to-control epilepsy patients.

The U.S. Food and Drug Administration permits generic bioavailability to vary between 80 percent and 125 percent from the brand-name medication. Bioavailability can also vary among generics for the same AED.

One can envision a circumstance in which a patient switches from Tegretol to a generic carbamazepine, with a resultant drop in levels of 20 percent. When that prescription runs out, the patient receives a generic at the pharmacy from a different manufacturer, which results in an increase of 25 percent relative to the original Tegretol, or a 45 percent increase from the previous generic. Although some patients may tolerate plasma level fluctuations of this degree, patients who are sensitive to side effects or have recurrent seizures are unlikely to benefit from generic medications. One trip to the ER for a breakthrough seizure can eliminate years of cost savings from generic medication.

Generic medications provide a useful alternative for patients whose seizures are easily controlled, take few if any other medications, and cannot afford brand-name AEDs. If patients do take a generic medication, they should try to stay with the same manufacturer.

38. When should I order a free antiepileptic drug level?

Free levels are important when serum protein binding is altered.

Paradoxically, "free" levels cost approximately twice as much as standard AED levels. The free level represents the unbound, active portion of the AED. Standard laboratory techniques measure total (bound and unbound) AED concentrations. Under normal circumstances, it is unnecessary to measure the free level because it represents a predictable percentage of the total drug. However, certain situations affect the ratio of free and bound drug:

- Hyperbilirubinemia
- Pregnancy
- Hypoalbuminemia
- Renal failure
- Hepatic failure
- Presence of other protein-bound drugs, including AEDs

When patients with these clinical situations continue to have seizures or experience AED toxicity, a free level provides better information on the amount of circulating active drug.

The free fraction of an AED may be elevated and neurotoxic despite a total drug concentration that is within the therapeutic range. For example, drug toxicity may occur when valproate is added to phenytoin. Patients typically attribute their symptoms to valproate, the newly added drug. In this case, valproate displaces phenytoin from its binding sites, causing an increase in the free phenytoin level and phenytoin toxicity. Standard AED measurement would not reveal this interaction.

39. Do antiepileptic drugs all work the same way?

No. Several pharmacologic strategies have been identified.

It probably is safe to say that we are not exactly certain how antiepileptic drugs (AEDs) prevent seizures. However, there appear to be at least five basic mechanisms of action. Most drugs fall into one or more of these categories.

1. Drugs that decrease sustained high-frequency repetitive firing of neurons by delaying recovery of sodium channels. Carbamazepine and phenytoin are classic examples of this mechanism. Lamotrigine's efficacy also appears due to voltage- and frequency-dependent inhibition of the sodium channel.
2. Drugs that reduce low-threshold (T-type) calcium channels. Ethosuximide, which is effective for absence seizures, is an example from this group.

3. Drugs that enhance gamma-aminobutyric acid (GABA) inhibition by acting on GABA receptor channels. Even within this group, strategies at the receptor differ. Barbiturates lengthen the duration of channel opening, whereas benzodiazepines increase the frequency of channel opening.
4. Drugs that enhance GABA by interfering with its inactivation, causing a relative excess of this inhibitory neurotransmitter. Tiagabine blocks the uptake of GABA from the synapse into presynaptic neurons and glial cells, increasing the amount of GABA in the synaptic cleft.
5. Drugs that inhibit neuroexcitation. Topiramate blocks kainate-evoked currents on the kainate/AMPA (a-amino-3-hydroxy-5-methylisoxazole-4-propionic acid) subtype of glutamate receptors.

Drugs can have more than one mechanism of action. Topiramate blocks sodium channels and enhances GABA. In addition, it is a carbonic anhydrase inhibitor and decreases calcium currents through high voltage–activated calcium channels. The relative contributions of these actions toward seizure control are not known.

Extensive research continues to lead to the development of novel compounds. Results are not always predictable. Gabapentin, which was designed to function as a GABA agonist, instead appears to increase intracellular GABA by an as yet undefined mechanism.

Understanding the mechanisms of AEDs allows one to pair them in a rational manner. For example, one can add a GABA enhancer such as tiagabine, which inhibits GABA reuptake, to a sodium channel blocker such as phenytoin, for additional effect. Our limited knowledge of mechanisms of action, as well as the problem of combined side effects, currently limits the benefits of polytherapy.

To further complicate matters, some AEDs, including carbamazepine and primidone, have one or more active metabolites. When treating a patient with one of these medications, even monotherapy becomes polytherapy!

Basic research continues to address the problem of controlling seizures by examining the cellular mechanisms involved in the epileptic discharge. The Anticonvulsant Screening Project at the University of Utah has screened thousands of potential antiepileptic compounds since it began in 1975. In addition, many scientists explore strategies to prevent or reverse brain conditions that allow the development of epilepsy. Potential targets for new AEDs include potassium channels, neurosteroid receptors, metabotropic receptors that generate second messengers, adenosine receptors, neurotrophin receptors, protein kinases, and gene expression.

5

Epilepsy and Pregnancy

When Janet and her husband arrived at my office for her first visit, she appeared visibly distraught. At first I thought her problem was poor seizure control. Each month she had five to six partial complex seizures and one convulsion. Her seizures continued despite therapeutic levels of phenytoin and divalproex sodium. She had seen a number of neurologists but had no luck trying phenobarbital, carbamazepine, or gabapentin.

Janet had meningitis at age 5 years, and her seizures began later that year. She had mild developmental delay and struggled through high school. College proved too difficult and she dropped out after only six months. She had trouble staying employed because of her seizures, inability to drive, and lack of job skills. She has, however, worked successfully as a housekeeper for the last three years.

Apart from her limited cognitive skills, neurologic examination was normal. Her electroencephalogram (EEG) showed left-sided slowing and occasional spikes. A computed axial tomography (CAT) scan was normal.

She married five years ago, at age 25. Her husband wants to have children. Janet said she had been trying to conceive for almost two years. She wasn't sure it was a good idea for her to have a child even if she could. She worried that her baby might have birth defects or epilepsy. Would it be better not to take any medication at all? Would she be able to safely care for the baby with her seizures? Wouldn't the medicines affect her child if she tried to breast-feed? Were the new

---

Note: See Resource R for a quick summary of recommendations for women with epilepsy and pregnancy.

*medications safer? Janet reached for her husband's hand. She stam-
mered and asked me whether I thought they should have a child.*

Questions

40. Should Janet have a baby?

Sure.

There are 20,000 births to women with epilepsy in the United States
every year. Most of the children are normal.

Whether any couple should have children is certainly up for discussion. Even if Janet did not have epilepsy, there still is a 2 percent
to 3 percent risk of congenital malformations, not to mention a lifetime of financial and emotional interdependence. There are a number
of additional considerations for a woman with uncontrolled seizures,
but none so great as to categorically rule out childbearing. As I discussed these issues with Janet and her husband, I made it clear that
the decision to have a child would be theirs, not mine. Let's look at
the issues.

41. Should Janet stop antiepileptic drugs?

No.

Even though Janet has frequent seizures and it appears that her
antiepileptic drugs (AEDs) are not helping, this is not the case. Without AEDs, Janet would probably have more frequent and more severe
seizures, as well as episodes of potentially life-threatening status
epilepticus.

Partial simple, partial complex, and absence seizures are not known
to increase the risk of fetal loss or injury. However, when a woman's
consciousness is altered during partial complex seizures, she may
become injured as a result of falls or burns. Trauma may threaten the
pregnancy.

Fetal bradycardia has been documented after a maternal convulsion,
suggesting fetal and maternal hypoxia and acidosis. Tonic-clonic
seizures can cause fetal intracranial hemorrhage and death. Status
epilepticus carries a 30 percent to 50 percent risk of mortality for the
unborn.

Risks of fetal and maternal injury must be weighed against the
potential teratogenesis of the AEDs. The American Academy of Neurology Quality Standards Subcommittee Practice Parameter (AAN

QSS)[1] recommends considering discontinuation of AEDs if a woman has been seizure-free for two to five years, has a single seizure type, a normal neurologic examination and IQ, and a normal EEG. In this situation, the woman should stop medications at least six months before conception to ensure that seizures will not recur during gestation.

Risk factors for relapse after AED withdrawal include a genetic syndrome such as juvenile myoclonic epilepsy, an abnormal magnetic resonance imaging study, and a history of status epilepticus.

42. Isn't there a risk of birth defects from antiepileptic drugs?

Yes.

As mentioned in answer 40, there is a risk of birth defects even without AEDs. The malformation rate in children of women with epilepsy is 1.5 to 2.5 times greater than that of the general population, or a risk of 4 percent to 8 percent. These birth defects include congenital heart disease, cleft lip and/or palate, neural tube defects (NTDs), genitourinary malformations, and limb defects. Although no randomized controlled studies relate congenital malformations and AEDs, a large part of this increased risk of congenital malformations is believed to be secondary to AEDs. All the commonly used AEDs—carbamazepine, ethosuximide, phenobarbital, phenytoin, primidone, and valproic acid—are known teratogens. The effects of the newer AEDs in the human fetus are not known.

Constellations of birth defects have been reported for the major AEDs, such as the fetal hydantoin syndrome, primidone embryopathy, carbamazepine syndrome, and valproic acid syndrome. Significant overlap occurs in these syndromes, and they are now lumped together as the "fetal AED syndrome."

Two AEDs are known to increase the risk of NTDs. Carbamazepine is associated with a 0.5–1% risk and valproic acid a 1–2% risk. NTDs result in birth defects, such as spina bifida and anencephaly. They occur because the neural tube fails to close properly between the third and fourth weeks of gestation.

The AAN QSS advises against changing AEDs during pregnancy if seizures are controlled in order to avoid exposing the fetus to more than one potential teratogen and risking seizure recurrence. Taking AEDs at lower doses more frequently throughout the day lowers peak levels and has a theoretical protective advantage.

One obstetrician called me about a women with well-controlled seizures who had recently conceived while taking gabapentin. The

---

[1] *Neurology* 1998;51:944–948

obstetrician insisted that I see her and switch her to a more conventional medication, such as phenobarbital or phenytoin, because the teratogenic risks of gabapentin were not known.

As long as the patient was seizure-free, I had considerable reluctance to switch to another AED and risk a breakthrough seizure. Neither did it make sense to expose the fetus to yet another drug. Nor could I agree with the logic that it was better to treat the patient with a known teratogen, such as phenobarbital or phenytoin, than with a new medication that may not be teratogenic at all!

Mechanisms of AED teratogenicity are not known. One hypothesis is that toxic intermediary metabolites rather than the parent compound cause the problems. Embryonic nucleic acid development may be disrupted by these reactive oxidative metabolites. Because gabapentin has no known metabolites, there is theoretical ground to suggest that it would be safe in pregnancy. More data about AEDs and teratogenic mechanisms must become available before a truly rational AED protocol for pregnancy exists. This work is under way.[2]

Socioeconomic and hereditary factors of women with epilepsy also contribute to the risk of teratogenesis, but these risk factors are less amenable to modification than are changes in AEDs.

On the other hand, despite the risks of heredity, socioeconomic factors, and AEDs, more than 90 percent of babies born to women with epilepsy will be normal.

43. Can the risk of congenital malformations be minimized?

Yes!

Several interventions may be helpful.

First, some women were placed on an antiepileptic drug (AED) as teenagers because of suspicious clinical events of passing out or "seizures," without a definite diagnosis. If this is the case, efforts should be made to confirm the diagnosis or withdraw the AED before conception.

Second, high AED levels are more damaging to the fetus than are low levels. Consequently, drug levels should be measured before conception, and the lowest effective AED dose prescribed. Repeat levels each trimester.

Third, polytherapy is worse than monotherapy. Multiple medications increase the risk of teratogenesis. Whenever possible, one AED should be used rather than two or three.

---

[2] An AED pregnancy registry has been established at Massachusetts General Hospital Genetics and Teratology Unit to try to learn more about teratogenesis and epilepsy. Women who become pregnant while taking AEDs should call toll-free 1-888-233-2334 to enroll in the registry and participate in three telephone interviews.

Janet's situation is difficult because she clearly has epilepsy and continues to have frequent seizures despite therapeutic levels of two AEDs. I would ask Janet to postpone her attempts at conception for at least several months and to try one or two of the newer AEDs, such as lamotrigine, oxcarbazepine, or topiramate. If she had a seizure reduction, I would aim for monotherapy[3] to reduce the risk of teratogenesis caused by polytherapy.

44. Can vitamins help?

Yes.

Low folate levels have been associated with fetal malformations in animal models and humans. Folate is a cofactor for the enzyme methionine synthetase, which is required for DNA biosynthesis. Carbamazepine, phenobarbital, and phenytoin can impair folate absorption. Consequently, there is a rationale for supplementing folate before and during pregnancy.

In addition, the literature supports folic acid supplementation to limit NTDs. Valproic acid is associated with a 1 percent to 2 percent risk of NTDs, and carbamazepine with a 0.5 percent to 1 percent risk. Valproic acid does not impair folate absorption, but rather inhibits glutamate formyl transferase, which prevents the conversion of folic acid to its active metabolite, folinic acid.

The Centers for Disease Control and Prevention recommend a dosage of 0.4 mg/day for primary prevention of NTDs in all women of childbearing age, regardless of whether they have epilepsy. Extrapolations from research in nonepileptic women suggest that dietary folate supplementation, up to 5 mg/day, may be protective.

There are no outcome studies that prove that folic acid supplementation in women with epilepsy prevents birth defects. However, folic acid supplementation seems worthwhile because there is indirect evidence that it may be helpful and because folic acid is inexpensive and innocuous at prescribed doses. A dose of 1–4 mg/day for women taking any AED, 4 mg/day for carbamazepine and valproate, is probably appropriate.

45. Is there prenatal testing for early detection of birth defects?

Yes.

A maternal alpha fetoprotein at 16 to 18 weeks will detect 85 percent of all open NTDs. An amniocentesis measuring both amniotic fluid

---

[3] As of this writing, lamotrigine and oxcarbazepine have been approved for monotherapy, but topiramate has not. However, prescribing medications for a woman in anticipation of pregnancy is a situation in which the potential benefits of monotherapy appear to warrant its use.

alpha fetoprotein and acetylcholinesterase is predictive of an open fetal NTD in more than 99 percent of cases. A structural ultrasound can detect NTDs and many other malformations. These tests can be performed early enough to consider termination of pregnancy. A thorough search for an NTD should be performed in women who conceived while taking carbamazepine or valproic acid.

The argument sometimes is made that there is no point in performing prenatal tests if a woman categorically refuses termination of pregnancy. However, early detection of significant fetal abnormalities can help the obstetrician plan a safer delivery. In addition, when faced with the reality of a catastrophic birth defect, some women will change their minds.

46. Should a woman take folic acid before she becomes pregnant?

Yes.

Approximately 40 percent of pregnancies in the United States are unplanned. Neural tube defects, which cause devastating birth defects such as spina bifida and anencephaly, occur because the neural tube fails to close properly between the third and fourth weeks of gestation. Consequently, NTDs occur before the mother is even aware of the pregnancy.

To prevent NTDs with folate supplementation, therefore, all women of childbearing age, whether contemplating pregnancy or not, should take this vitamin, as described in answer 44.

47. If Janet decides to postpone conception, should she use the birth control pill?

Probably not.

Many options exist for birth control, including barrier methods such as condoms and diaphragms, spermicidal foam, oral contraceptives, intrauterine contraceptive devices, levonorgestrel implants (Norplant), and hormonal injections.

Because many common AEDs (carbamazepine, oxcarbazepine, phenobarbital, phenytoin, primidone, and topiramate) induce enzymes of the cytochrome P450 system, oral hormonal contraceptive methods may not work as well. I have seen women become pregnant while taking AEDs and the birth control pill, as well as while using Norplant. (These women are *not* happy.)

If a woman chooses to use the birth control pill while taking an enzyme-inducing AED, the minimal dose of ethinyl estradiol or mestranol should be at least 50 µg. (Most oral contraceptives contain 35 µg of estrogen or less.) A barrier method provides additional protection.

Gabapentin, lamotrigine, levetiracetam, tiagabine, and valproic acid are not enzyme-inducers and do not require altering oral contraceptive dose.

48. Will oral contraceptives increase Janet's seizure frequency?

No.

There is much experimental evidence that ovarian steroids affect seizure susceptibility. Estrogens activate epileptiform discharges and may cause seizures. Estradiol increases synaptic excitability and increases the number of dendritic spines on hippocampal neurons in rat preparations. Estradiol facilitates kindled seizures in the amygdala and hippocampus. It lowers the seizure threshold for electroshock-induced seizures and kainic acid–induced seizures.

Progesterone has the opposite effect—decreasing neuronal firing and epileptiform discharges and increasing the seizure threshold in animal models.

The occurrence of seizures in some women in temporal relation to the monthly period (catamenial epilepsy) supports this relationship of gonadal hormones and seizures. Nonetheless, there is no convincing clinical evidence that birth control pills affect seizure frequency.

49. But Janet hasn't used any birth control at all for two years. Does epilepsy affect fertility?

Yes.

Janet and her husband suffer from infertility, which is defined as the failure to conceive after one year of intercourse without contraception. Fertility in women with epilepsy is reduced by up to 85 percent as compared with the general population and 37 percent less than family controls. Partial seizures and an early age of seizure onset are predictors for low fertility. Many women with epilepsy have abnormal menstrual cycles, which may be due to lack of ovulation or to insufficient progesterone secretion in the luteal phase.

As many as 35 percent of women with temporal lobe epilepsy have anovulatory cycles. Women with epilepsy may develop polycystic ovaries, and polycystic ovary syndrome (PCOS) is increased fourfold in women with temporal lobe epilepsy. Women with temporal lobe epilepsy and PCOS have increased luteinizing hormone (LH) pulse frequency and may be more likely to have left-sided epileptic activity. The incidence of hypothalamic hypogonadism (HH) also is increased in women with temporal lobe epilepsy. Anovulatory cycles occur in both PCOS and HH.

Epilepsy may affect hormonal control because of extensive connections between the mesial temporal lobe structures and the hypothalamus. Infertility in women with epilepsy may be related to epileptic discharges, which disrupt hypothalamic hormone release and affect the hypothalamic-pituitary axis. An abnormal pituitary response to gonadotropin-releasing hormone (GnRH), altered release of LH, abnormal concentrations of pituitary LH, and increased pituitary prolactin may occur. Twenty-five percent to 65 percent of women with temporal lobe epilepsy have decreased libido and difficulty in achieving orgasm. Women with epilepsy also are more likely to suffer physiologic sexual dysfunction such as vaginismus, dyspareunia, and arousal insufficiency. These symptoms can contribute to infertility.

Women should see a specialist in fertility or a gynecologist if they have intermenstrual bleeding, bleeding lasting more than seven days, periods occurring at intervals of three weeks or less or more than 35 days apart, or inability to conceive after one year. Most patients with epilepsy are able to conceive.

50. If Janet finally does conceive, is it likely that her baby will have epilepsy too?

No.

Most women of childbearing age with epilepsy suffer from idiopathic epilepsy, seizures of unknown cause. Other common epilepsy etiologies in this age group are head trauma, encephalitis, meningitis, and birth defects. Epilepsy related to a genetic cause likely to be passed on to children, such as juvenile myoclonic epilepsy or absence epilepsy, constitutes a minority of cases. Even when there is a genetic cause, the inheritance pattern is rarely autosomal dominant, and the child is more likely to be healthy than to have epilepsy. Overall, the risk of a mother with epilepsy giving birth to a baby who will develop epilepsy is approximately 3 percent.

51. Is Janet more likely to have obstetric and perinatal complications?

Probably.

Pregnant women with epilepsy are best managed in a high-risk obstetric clinic, such as is common for women with diabetes. Although there is inconsistency in the studies, there are reports of higher rates of spontaneous abortion, preeclampsia, maternal bleeding, hyperemesis gravidarum, premature labor and preterm delivery, forceps or vacuum-assisted delivery, caesarean section, stillbirth, and perinatal death.

The advantage of a high-risk clinic is the increased vigilance for these problems and the more frequent and focused attention on the patient's seizures, AED levels, and psychosocial stresses. In my practice, I found that compliance with visits to the high-risk clinic was far greater than in my office, which suggests that most women with epilepsy appreciate the importance of prenatal care. This provides the physician with nine months of close follow-up for refining the diagnosis and treatment.

52. Do some women have an increase in seizure frequency during pregnancy?

Yes.

Approximately one third of women experience increased seizures during pregnancy. Lowered AED levels may occur as a result of vomiting or decreased absorption. The woman may stop taking the medication because of fears of birth defects. Increased hepatic blood flow and renal clearance also decrease AED levels. Increased neuroactive ovarian hormone levels may lower the seizure threshold. If seizures do occur, the possibility of eclampsia should also be kept in mind.

Approximately 1 percent to 2 percent of women with epilepsy have a convulsion at the time of delivery. Sleep deprivation, stress, and low serum levels of AEDs may contribute. A seizure in the delivery room can be treated with a benzodiazepine if necessary. Antiepileptic drug levels should be checked when the woman presents in labor.

Decreased protein binding of AEDs related to reduced serum albumin and competition for binding sites from sex steroid hormones results in lower measured AED levels, although the nonbound (free) fraction may not be similarly reduced. For highly bound medications, such as carbamazepine, phenytoin, and valproic acid, free AED levels more accurately represent the active levels in the central nervous system.

53. Are any other vitamins helpful?

Yes.

In addition to prenatal vitamins, vitamin K1 may help reduce neonatal hemorrhagic complications that occur within the first 24 hours of birth. Antiepileptic drugs that induce the cytochrome P450 enzyme system can result in decreased vitamin K, vitamin K-dependent clotting factors, prolonged partial thromboplastin time, and prothrombin time. These deficits may produce coagulopathy and neonatal hemorrhage. To prevent these problems, prescribe oral vitamin K1, 10 mg/day, beginning at 36 weeks gestation.

54. Is breast-feeding recommended?

Yes.

Antiepileptic drugs are secreted in breast milk. The more protein-bound they are, the less they are secreted. Some neonates may reach therapeutic levels of AEDs because of breast milk ingestion. Reports of idiosyncratic drug toxicity from AEDs are exceedingly rare. There is one report of methemoglobinemia related to phenytoin and another report of thrombocytopenic purpura and anemia secondary to valproic acid. More commonly, an infant may become sedated from a barbiturate.

There are nutritional and immunologic advantages to breast-feeding. Breast-feeding should be continued if the infant appears alert and is able to suck. If the mother is taking barbiturates, one should carefully observe the infant for withdrawal symptoms when breast-feeding is terminated.

55. Will Janet be able to care for the baby?

She will need help.

Six partial complex seizures per month will place the baby's health at risk. If Janet has an alteration of consciousness while changing, bathing, or carrying the infant, the results could be disastrous. She will need to learn to minimize risks, such as changing the baby on the floor rather than on a changing table, bathing the baby only when accompanied by another adult, and carrying the baby as little as possible. Janet's husband, parents, and in-laws will all have to participate in the care of the infant. A social worker may be able to find community services.

One of my patients with intractable epilepsy and poor memory had very limited resources and no family support but desperately wanted to keep her baby. The social worker was able to connect with her local church and obtained enormous assistance. The neighborhood church community effectively adopted her and the baby as a special project. Volunteers provided almost 24-hour-a-day live-in help.

Delivering a healthy baby is just the beginning. . . .

6

Rash!

Tony flashed a glittering smile as he glided into my cramped office for a second opinion. He had just come from his job as floor manager at the BMW dealership and looked sharp in his three-piece suit and waxed handlebar mustache. This 40-year-old man wanted to know if he could stop taking his phenytoin. He seemed bright and interested as we reviewed his case together.

Gestation was uneventful, but he appeared jaundiced at birth. He experienced his first seizure at age 7 months. There was no fever. He took phenobarbital and had several more afebrile seizures over the next year. His last childhood seizure occurred at age 18 months. His pediatrician finally discontinued phenobarbital when Tony graduated from high school.

Tony did fine without medication for the next 24 years. But on March 12, 1998, he developed a headache severe enough to bring him to the community hospital. He was prescribed a painkiller and an antibiotic for a sinus infection and was sent home. Six days later, he shocked his coworkers with a grand mal seizure in the showroom. An ambulance returned him to the hospital, where he had a second convulsion. After a computed axial tomographic (CAT) scan and a lumbar puncture, he was diagnosed with acute sinusitis, meningitis, and orbital cellulitis with a subperiosteal orbital abscess.

Tony received antibiotics for six weeks in hospital and had a right external ethmoidectomy. Because of his meningitis and the two convulsions, he was loaded with phenytoin and kept on a maintenance dose. He had no further seizures.

Now, five months later, he wants to know if he still needs the anticonvulsant. Since his discharge from the hospital, he has noticed problems with his memory and trouble controlling his emotions. He told me he was short-tempered by nature, but that it was worse now. He recently blew up at a coworker over who would be the first to read the sports pages in the newspaper. He realized that his reaction was inappropriate but told me he couldn't control himself.

He complains of daily headaches, which last from an hour to all day. They are accompanied by photophobia but no fever, nausea, or vomiting. Aspirin sometimes helps. He feels slightly fatigued after he takes his morning dose of phenytoin, but then improves. He also has noted a variable tremor in both hands.

He has had recurrent bouts of sinusitis since discharge from the hospital. His oral surgeon prescribes antibiotics over the phone. During these episodes his head feels full and he has a nasal discharge.

His past medical history is remarkable for a myocardial infarction two years ago and mild arthritis. His only medications are phenytoin, 300 mg/day, and an occasional aspirin. He has smoked at least two packs of cigarettes a day for as long as he can remember. He occasionally drinks alcohol. No one in his family has epilepsy.

His medical examination was normal. Despite complaints of decreased memory and irritability, his mental status also was normal. Neurologic examination revealed a bilateral postural and intention tremor, left greater than right.

Tony didn't have any current imaging studies, but his CAT scan from the hospital was fairly impressive. There was erosion of the right maxillary wall, a right orbital abscess, sinusitis, right frontal cerebritis, and an epidural abscess on the right frontal lobe. A magnetic resonance imaging study showed similar findings, as well as proptosis of the right eye and right frontal lobe edema. An electroencephalogram (EEG) revealed independent slowing and sharp waves in both temporal regions.

I told Tony that, given his history of childhood seizures, combined with his recent meningitis, cerebritis, frontal lobe edema, emotional lability, and abnormal EEG, it was prudent to continue his phenytoin for now. Maybe we could stop it in a few years if he remained seizure-free. I suggested that we check a phenytoin level to make sure he was getting enough and that he wasn't toxic. I thought a repeat EEG might shed some light on how his brain was recovering. I reminded him that less cigarette smoke would also be to his advantage.

Tony took the news well, satisfied that someone had given his situation some thought. He made an appointment for a checkup in six months. I was confident with my assessment, delighted to have a pleasant patient with a straightforward problem.

Two days later I got a call from an emergency room (ER) 50 miles away, where Tony worked. The ER doctor described a rash around Tony's eyes, forehead, and malar regions. The skin was slightly indurated and tender.

Mild edema distorted his eyelids. According to Tony, it was itchy and felt like a "flashburn." There were no lesions on his lips or tongue. His temperature was 100°F. There was blood when he blew his nose. Tony thought that maybe he was getting sinusitis again. The ER doctor gave him some diphenhydramine and wanted to send him home with antibiotics.

I asked him to discontinue the phenytoin because of a possible allergic reaction and to begin gabapentin. I insisted that Tony see me in clinic the next day. I also arranged for him to have another CAT scan of his sinuses to clarify whether he had recurrent sinusitis.

Questions

56. Are rashes common with antiepileptic drugs?

Yes.

Rashes have been a problem ever since bromine was used as the first modern anticonvulsant in 1857. Bromides cause an acneiform rash on the face that may spread to the rest of the body, as well as vesicles, pustules, and ulcerations.

I recently gave a lecture and asked a room of 100 or so neurologists how many of them had seen a phenytoin rash. All of them raised their hands. I repeated the question substituting carbamazepine and the same hands went up again. When I asked about valproate, approximately three quarters of the audience raised their hands.

One report from the neurosurgical literature described a 19 percent incidence of rash in patients with head trauma treated with phenytoin. Although they were followed up for almost four years, all the rashes occurred between Days 5 and 91. Most were morbilliform (measles-like, for those of you who remember that disease) rashes. One patient had an exfoliative dermatitis, and one had a pseudolymphoma type syndrome.

Approximately 10 percent of patients taking carbamazepine experience a hypersensitivity rash, especially during the first weeks or months. These risks compare with 1 percent to 3 percent of patients who have allergic reactions to cephalosporin drugs.

57. Did I need to stop Tony's phenytoin?

Probably not.

The redness and swelling in Tony's face was most likely caused by recurrent sinusitis. But I was concerned about a drug allergy, and possibly a rare, severe drug reaction called anticonvulsant hypersensitivity syndrome (AHS).

Anticonvulsant hypersensitivity syndrome occurs in 1 of 3,000 antiepileptic drug (AED) exposures. Synonyms are the Dilantin hypersensitivity syndrome, phenytoin/Dilantin syndrome, Kawasaki-like syndrome, hypersensitivity to aromatic anticonvulsant agents, and mononucleosis-like syndrome. The triad of fever, skin rash, and internal organ involvement characterizes AHS.

In general, symptoms occur two to eight weeks after AED initiation. The liver is involved in more than one half of cases, followed by eosinophilia, blood dyscrasias, nephritis, lung involvement, and atypical lymphocytosis. Patients may also have pharyngitis, facial angioedema, and lymphadenopathy. The aromatic AEDs—phenytoin, carbamazepine, phenobarbital, and primidone—usually cause this syndrome.

The etiology is not known, but it may be related to a toxic arene oxide metabolite of the aromatic AEDs. Anticonvulsant hypersensitivity syndrome can be confused with mononucleosis, viral hepatitis, toxic shock syndrome, systemic lupus erythematosus, and other systemic illnesses. Mortality can reach 20 percent.

Tony's facial angioedema probably was due to his sinusitis, but it also could have been related to AHS. Anticonvulsant hypersensitivity syndrome was less likely because the rash was confined to his face and he felt well. On the other hand, he had a slight fever, again probably caused by his sinusitis, but possibly related to a systemic drug reaction. Blood tests looking for hepatitis, leukopenia, eosinophilia, and atypical lymphocytosis would have been helpful. But even had they all been normal, I still would have stopped the phenytoin. (It's always a judgment call.)

58. I'm a neurologist, not a dermatologist. Can I tell a drug rash from the myriad of other rashes?

Often.

The first step is to get a history, then see the rash. Because patients are warned about possible skin eruptions when starting a new medication, they often find them. It may be impossible to diagnose the cause of a skin rash over the telephone. I have had patients complain of allergic reactions to AEDs when they suffered from flea bites, fungal infections, or acne, all of which were fairly obvious on examination.

The typical drug reaction begins as a morbilliform or exanthematous rash. It may be pruritic. Prominent on the chest and back, it may spread to the extremities and face. A drug rash usually occurs within the first six months of treatment. A patient who has been taking phenytoin for 10 years is unlikely to develop a spontaneous allergic rash. Because

Tony had been taking phenytoin for five months, a drug rash, although not likely, was still a reasonable consideration.

Here are diagnostic features of four other illnesses that are important in the differential diagnosis of rash. These diseases require prompt and specific treatment, and must be distinguished from a drug reaction.

- Rocky Mountain spotted fever, which is transmitted by a tick, occurs primarily in the south central and southeastern United States, particularly during the spring and summer. The rash usually begins on Day 4 of the illness and begins on the ankles and wrists, spreading to the soles and palms and then to the torso. This pattern is very different from a drug rash, which typically begins on the torso. However, once the rash has spread, it may resemble a drug rash.
- Meningococcal infection, which is caused by an encapsulated gram-negative diplococcus, occurs primarily in the winter and spring in children and young adults. The characteristic skin rash is a diffuse petechial eruption that evolves into pathognomonic palpable purpura with gunmetal gray necrotic centers. Macular, papular, and urticarial lesions may develop. Petechiae tend to cluster at areas of pressure. Skin findings are more common in children. Purpura fulminans can occur if the disease advances to Waterhouse-Friderichsen syndrome with disseminated intravascular coagulation; it is characterized by large ecchymoses and hemorrhagic bullae.
- Staphylococcal toxic shock syndrome, which originally was associated with tampon use, but also is seen from wound infections, nasal packing, and other localized staphylococcal infections, produces prominent symptoms of fever, malaise, nausea, and confusion. The skin initially appears reddened as if by sunburn, followed by desquamation, especially of the hands and feet.
- Streptococcal toxic shock syndrome, which is caused by production of group A streptococcus pyrogenic exotoxins, produces erythema and tenderness. Violaceous bullae occur if the infection advances to necrotizing fasciitis.

A directed history looking for possible infectious exposure or contact with skin irritants may help exclude causes other than drugs. Constitutional symptoms such as fever, lymphadenopathy, and malaise suggest a systemic illness or severe drug reaction. A physical examination looking for mucosal lesions, lymphadenopathy, signs of hepatitis, edema, and other systemic abnormalities will also aid in diagnosis.

59. Can I tell a serious drug rash from a benign one?

Yes (but usually when it's too late)!

Unfortunately, serious allergic rashes typically start out looking just like benign rashes. This phenomenon creates a quandary in the medical management of a so-called benign-looking rash. Approximately 50 percent of drug rashes will diminish after lowering the AED dose or stopping it, permitting the patient to continue or restart the medication. However, the other half will not. Consequently, it is very difficult to give a blanket recommendation on what to do when a patient develops a drug rash. A dermatology consultation may be helpful.

Patients with a serious, potentially life-threatening rash develop systemic signs such as fever, malaise, arthralgia, myalgia, and lymphadenopathy. Papules, vesicles, target lesions, erosions, and desquamation characterize the more severe drug rashes such as anticonvulsant hypersensitivity syndrome (AHS), erythema multiforme, Stevens-Johnson syndrome (SJS), and toxic epidermal necrolysis (TEN).

A painful or burning rash is ominous. Tony described his rash as a "flashburn," which heightened my level of concern. Similarly, angioedema, particularly of the face and around the eyes, portends a systemic and potentially severe reaction. A positive Nikolsky's sign, in which lateral pressure easily separates the outer epidermis from the basal skin layer, indicates a serious cutaneous reaction.

Laboratory studies in AHS may reveal eosinophilia, atypical lymphocytosis, hepatitis, leukopenia, nephritis, thrombocytopenia, and hemolytic anemia.

Involvement of mucous membranes suggests SJS, which has a 10 percent mortality. The mortality of TEN, which is characterized by greater than 30 percent of epidermal detachment, is even higher.

60. Do I always have to stop the antiepileptic drug when a patient develops a rash?

No.

Many of my colleagues try to ride out a drug rash by lowering the dose and vigilant observation. I almost always stop the drug. The risk of a severe systemic illness, superimposed on my patient's epilepsy, is usually too great a threat to continue the medication. I make exceptions when the patient has had a remarkable therapeutic response to a particular AED while having dismal failures from others. In other words, if the patient has few options left, I may try to proceed with the offending drug by lowering the dose and carefully monitoring the patient's progress, at least daily. This approach also requires a compliant patient who will return regularly for reassessment.

I stop the drug immediately if the patient has any systemic signs, such as fever, wheezing, or malaise. A blistering rash or skin detachment also forces drug discontinuation. Most of the time, I try an alternate drug and hope the rash goes away.

If the patient's seizures are infrequent, I often wait a few days until the rash begins to disappear before initiating a replacement drug. Otherwise, if the rash persists or worsens during the introduction of the new AED, it raises the question of an allergy to the second drug as well.

61. Is there cross-reactivity between some of the antiepileptic drugs?

Yes.

Carbamazepine, phenytoin, and phenobarbital, all with arene ring chemical structures, demonstrate cross-reactivity as high as 80 percent for AHS. Consequently, if a patient develops a drug rash with carbamazepine or phenytoin, it is best to choose another medication, such as valproate, gabapentin, or topiramate, which have different structures and a lower incidence of rashes.

62. If a patient develops AHS with phenytoin, is it likely to occur with lamotrigine?

Maybe.

Lamotrigine, a phenyltriazine, belongs to a different class of AEDs than phenytoin. However, it has also been associated with anticonvulsant hypersensitivity syndrome. Consequently, it would be prudent to avoid lamotrigine in this setting.

In approximately 1 of 1,000 adults and 1 of 100 children, lamotrigine has been associated with potentially life-threatening reactions, including SJS and TEN. Rapid dosing or concomitant use of valproic acid, which prolongs the half-life of lamotrigine, are thought to increase the risk of rash. Most, but not all, cases of life-threatening rash with lamotrigine occur within two to eight weeks of treatment. In premarketing clinical trials, 0.3 percent of patients required hospitalization for a serious skin rash. Benign rashes also occur.

Rash of any type occurred in 10 percent of patients taking lamotrigine in clinical studies. Typically, maculopapular, morbilliform, or erythematous eruptions occur in the first four to six weeks. Rash is the most frequent single reason for patients terminating treatment with lamotrigine. In clinical trials, 3.8 percent of patients discontinued lamotrigine because of rash. Starting with a low dose and increasing by small increments may decrease the incidence of rash.

63. Are certain antiepileptic drugs unlikely to produce a rash?

Yes.

For example, rash with valproate occurs in approximately 6 percent of exposures, less frequently than with phenytoin or carbamazepine. Anticonvulsant hypersensitivity syndrome rarely occurs with valproate. This may be related to structural differences between the compounds—valproate has a fatty acid structure and does not share a benzene ring.

Carbamazepine and phenytoin are metabolized by cytochrome P450 to an arene oxide metabolite. This metabolite is normally detoxified by epoxide hydrolase. It is postulated that patients who develop AHS may have an epoxide hydrolase deficiency.

To complicate matters, valproate inhibits epoxide hydrolase. Consequently, valproate may prolong the rash when used with aromatic AEDs.

Topiramate, one of the newer AEDs, has a reported incidence of rash similar to that of placebo. Rash also is uncommon with gabapentin, levetiracetam, oxcarbazepine, phenobarbital, and tiagabine.

64. Will routine blood monitoring predict an allergic hypersensitivity reaction?

No.

Clinical symptoms precede abnormal blood tests in cases of exfoliative dermatitis. Mild transaminase elevations or benign leukopenia do not predict more severe reactions.

65. Was gabapentin a good choice for Tony?

Yes.

I wanted to choose a drug with a low incidence of rash that I could dose rapidly. Gabapentin rarely causes allergic rash and can be increased to the maintenance dose within a few days. Although topiramate has a low incidence of rash, it may take several weeks to achieve therapeutic doses. Tiagabine also takes weeks to achieve full dosing. I did not know whether Tony had hepatitis to go along with his angioedema, so I avoided valproate, which can be hepatotoxic. Otherwise, valproate also would have been a reasonable choice.

Tony's sinus radiographs confirmed sinusitis, and his rash and facial swelling resolved after several days of antibiotics. Because he tolerated the gabapentin, I did not switch him back to phenytoin. I also did not want him to continue a medication that might compromise his showroom smile.

7

Epilepsy and Psychiatric Disorders

Donna is a 51-year-old woman with uncontrolled seizures. Gestation, birth, and development were normal. At the age of four years, she tumbled down a flight of stairs and was unconscious for less than a minute. She had her first seizure at age 6. Until recently all her seizures were staring spells. However, last year she began having "funny feelings" followed by episodes of wandering and confusion. Sometimes she suddenly becomes stiff and her arms jerk. Seizures occur at any time of day. She never has olfactory, auditory, or visual auras. There is no history of febrile seizures, myoclonic jerks, encephalitis, meningitis, or a family history of epilepsy.

Over the years Donna has tried carbamazepine, ethotoin, gabapentin, lamotrigine, phenobarbital, phenytoin, primidone, tiagabine, topiramate, and valproate, all without successful seizure control. She thinks she had some sort of "allergic" reaction to phenobarbital.

She complains of significant memory difficulties. Donna worked as a lab technician until five years ago, but she could no longer work unsupervised because of increasing seizures and attention problems. To pass the time, she spends every Sunday at church and attends bible study classes four evenings a week.

Several years ago she fractured her wrist in a seizure-related fall. Her family doctor noted a low leukocyte count, which he has been following. She has been evaluated in the emergency room (ER) several times for chest pain and paresthesias in both arms, but no cardiac disease has been detected.

She complains of feeling intoxicated and has trouble walking down stairs. She fell last week and hit her head on the front steps of her apartment. Six months ago she spent two weeks in a psychiatric hos-pital for depression and an intentional drug overdose.

She takes a combination of lamotrigine, phenytoin, and tiagabine, as well as clorazepate, estrogen, sertraline, and vitamin D. She doesn't smoke, drink, or abuse drugs. She is divorced with no children. She surrendered her driver's license after crashing into a parked car during a seizure. The accident occurred soon after she lost her job. Now she reluctantly depends on her sister for transportation.

Donna's sister, Mary, is a nurse practitioner. She came with her to the office and sat quietly, interjecting only when absolutely necessary. When I asked how often she had seizures, Donna began a rambling, tangential answer that lasted more than 10 minutes without coming to a conclusion. When I interrupted her, she became very upset, cried, and proclaimed that she never got to finish what she wanted to say and that no one ever listened to her. When her sister admonished her that she was exaggerating, Donna launched into a hurtful tirade, accusing her of meddling in her affairs and not letting her "be her own person."

When she finally calmed down, I performed a physical examination, which was normal apart from a mild bruise on her scalp. Although Donna was mildly hostile, she cooperated with the neurologic exami-nation. I found only a bilateral tremor and brisk reflexes.

A magnetic resonance imaging scan revealed right mesial temporal sclerosis. Right temporal spikes and slow waves were seen on a routine electroencephalogram several years ago.

Questions

66. Do all patients with epilepsy have psychiatric disorders?

No.

Uncontrolled epilepsy often leads to unemployment and loss of dri-ving privileges. These two problems result in loss of professional iden-tity, financial difficulties, and social isolation. In addition, physiologic factors such as memory loss, cognitive impairment, and ongoing epileptic activity contribute to a mood disorder.

Not all patients with epilepsy have psychiatric symptoms. However, mood changes, suicide attempts, and psychosis are more common in patients with epilepsy. More than half of chronic epilepsy patients admitted to the hospital for video-EEG monitoring require psychiatric intervention.

Behavior disorders result from interactions between the patient's genetic and constitutional makeup, the nature and location of brain injury causing the seizures, the intrinsic effects of the epileptic activity on the brain, the psychosocial environment, and antiepileptic and other medication therapy. Although the primary focus of a patient's doctor visit usually is seizure control, a careful behavioral history should be elicited to look for symptoms that may warrant treatment.

Concurrent psychiatric disorders can greatly complicate the treatment of patients with epilepsy. Some antiepileptic drugs cause behavior problems, often while reducing seizure frequency. Antidepressants and antipsychotic medications lower the seizure threshold, potentially exacerbating the seizure disorder. Treatment of two disorders often requires polytherapy, which raises the potential for drug-drug interactions. Psychiatric disease may impair compliance with doctor visits and medication regimens.

Behavior disorders can be classified as preictal, ictal, postictal, and interictal. Among other structures, the limbic system includes the hippocampus, parahippocampal gyrus, and amygdala—all prominent components of the temporal lobe. Consequently, it is not surprising that structural or electrical lesions of the temporal lobes can result in behavioral abnormalities of mood, affect, motivation, and sexual function. Subtle abnormalities, such as impaired facial recognition and inability to recognize the emotions of others, contribute to suboptimal interpersonal relationships.

67. What is the most common type of behavior disorder seen in epilepsy patients?

Mood disorder.

Mood disorder occurs far more frequently than psychosis. A specific type of mood disorder recently identified in epilepsy patients, interictal dysphoric disorder (IDD), requires antidepressant treatment in up to one half of patients with chronic epilepsy. Patients with temporal lobe epilepsy are at highest risk.

Eight symptoms characterize IDD: depressive mood, anergia, pain, insomnia, fear, anxiety, paroxysmal irritability, and euphoric moods. Depressive mood, anergia, and irritability occur most commonly. Unlike primary depression, whose symptoms tend to be persistent, perhaps improving over the course of a day, symptoms of IDD tend to be intermittent, lasting for hours or a few days and recurring at irregular intervals. Donna's symptoms of depressed mood, fear, anxiety, and paroxysmal irritability are consistent with IDD.

The physiologic cause of the mood disorder in patients with temporal lobe epilepsy is not clear. It tends to develop gradually in patients with chronic epilepsy and may become more pronounced when seizure activity is suppressed, which suggests that the mood disorder may result from inhibitory mechanisms that develop in response to epileptic activity. Positron emission tomography (PET) scans reveal hypometabolism, which extends beyond the temporal lobe into the thalamus and frontal lobes. Frontal lobe hypometabolism may be related to depression. The interictal hypometabolic zone also demonstrates enhanced opioid receptor binding.

68. Can interictal dysphoric disorder be treated?

Yes.

The most economical medication treatment for IDD is with a tricyclic antidepressant (TCA), such as imipramine, at a dose from 100 to 150 mg at bedtime. Clinical response occurs rapidly, often within days rather than weeks, with improvement not only in depressive symptoms (sleep, anergia, insomnia, pain), but also in irritability, fear, and anxiety. If patients do not respond, a selective serotonin reuptake inhibitor (SSRI) can be added. Paroxetine, venlafaxine, and sertraline probably are the safest. Antidepressants such as amoxapine, bupropion, clomipramine, and maprotiline should be avoided because they significantly lower the seizure threshold.

Several drug-drug interactions deserve mention. Selective serotonin reuptake inhibitors can increase TCA levels, fluoxetine can raise phenytoin levels, and fluoxetine and carbamazepine can cause serotonin syndrome.

If a patient has severe refractory major depression, electroshock therapy (ECT) can be safely used. Indications for ECT are the same as for patients without epilepsy.

Prudence in prescribing large quantities of medication is required for patients with depression. An overdose, particularly with TCAs, may be lethal.

Control of the epileptic seizures and reversal of work and driving limitations may also improve the patient's outlook.

69. Did antidepressant treatment make Donna's seizures worse?

Probably not.

Although antidepressants may exacerbate seizure disorders, a recent study revealed that most patients treated with antidepressants did not have an increase in seizure frequency, although 23 percent did. Tricyclic antidepressants lower the seizure threshold more than the SSRIs do. The effect of lithium on seizure frequency has been debated. The treatment of depression warrants the risk of seizure exacerbation in most instances.

Most patients with partial seizures have a stable clinical course over time. Some patients have improvement of their seizures, whereas others experience increased seizure frequency or severity. Donna's seizures now are more intense, with pronounced alteration of consciousness and some secondary generalization. Her cognitive and memory problems have become so severe that she can no longer work. Depression may adversely affect her memory and attention as well.

70. Can antiepileptic medications cause depression?

Yes.

Donna gave a vague history of an allergy to phenobarbital. Most likely she did not have a typical allergic reaction with a pruritic rash, which would be memorable, but rather an episode of depression with phenobarbital. In a study comparing patients treated with phenobarbital with patients receiving carbamazepine, 40 percent of the patients on phenobarbital had depressive disorder compared with only 4 percent of those on carbamazepine. In addition, 47 percent of the phenobarbital patients had suicidal ideation, compared with 4 percent of the carbamazepine patients.

Depression, suicidal ideation, attempted suicide, and successful suicide are increased in patients treated with phenobarbital. Phenobarbital should be used cautiously, if at all, in patients with a history of depression. Primidone also should be avoided because one of its metabolites is phenobarbital.

Clonazepam, felbamate, tiagabine, topiramate, and vigabatrin have all been associated with depression. Patients should be monitored carefully for depressive symptoms while taking these medications.

71. Is suicide a significant problem in patients with epilepsy?

Yes.

Suicide is four to five times more common in patients with epilepsy than in the general population. Patients with temporal lobe epilepsy may have a risk as great as 25 times what would be expected. Suicide attempts are also more common in patients with epilepsy. Other risk factors include psychiatric hospitalizations, alcohol and psychoactive substance abuse, antisocial and borderline personality disorders, primary affective disorder, schizophrenia, male gender, Caucasian race, living alone, poor physical health, and age over 45 years. In one study, barbiturates and hydantoin drug overdoses were the most common suicide method.

Suicide attempts may increase in frequency after improvement of seizure control. In one study, suicide was the most common cause of death after temporal lobectomy. Early recognition of mood disorder by health care professionals may diminish patient death from suicide.

Donna has uncontrolled seizures, one hospitalization for depression, and a suicide attempt. She currently is taking sertraline, an SSRI, for depression. She also is taking clorazepate, a benzodiazepine, probably for her anxiety. I encouraged her to follow up with her psychiatrist, as she is still clearly symptomatic despite medication treatment. She continues to be at high risk for suicide. The addition of a TCA might be helpful.

72. Are patients with epilepsy more susceptible to psychosis?

Yes.

Intractable epilepsy patients with multiple seizure types, long duration of epilepsy, and a history of status epilepticus are at greatest risk for developing psychosis. Psychosis is much more common in patients with temporal lobe epilepsy than extratemporal epilepsy. The mean interval between the onset of seizures and the onset of psychosis is 14 years. Psychosis is seen more often at epilepsy centers, which treat more severely affected patients. Depending on the epilepsy population, psychosis ranges widely from 2 percent to 60 percent. Epilepsy patients in psychiatric hospitals have the highest prevalence of psychosis.

The most frequent form of psychosis in epilepsy patients occurs interictally. Many observers believe that these symptoms differ from the psychosis of process schizophrenia with preservation of affect, fewer motor symptoms, and increased delusions and mystical religious experiences. Interictal epileptic psychosis also responds better to medication.

Antipsychotic medications may be necessary for symptomatic treatment. Patients taking antiepileptic drugs that are enzyme-inducers may need higher doses of antipsychotics. Like antidepressants, neuroleptic medications lower the seizure threshold. Butyrophenones are less likely to provoke seizures than are phenothiazines. Chlorpromazine should be avoided.

Of the newer antipsychotics, clozapine causes seizures in 2.8 percent of patients. Risperidone has only a 0.3 percent incidence of seizures and probably is the neuroleptic of choice for patients with both epilepsy and psychosis.

As a general guideline, one can reduce the risk of seizures by using low doses of neuroleptic medications and increasing doses slowly. Avoid combinations of neuroleptics.

Approximately 25 percent of psychoses in epileptic patients occur postictally. Patients often have a flurry of generalized tonic-clonic seizures from which they recover. However, after one to six days of a relatively lucid interval, they become psychotic, with hallucinations and severe abnormal behavior. One of my patients developed a postictal psychosis after having multiple seizures during video monitoring. She spent hours looking around her hospital room and smiling. She would say "hi," but few other words. Once she remarked that "the TV has gone away" and complained that her "teeth were falling out." Her psychotic symptoms disappeared after several days, and she demanded to know why she was still in the hospital.

Psychotic symptoms usually disappear within 14 days. Low doses of neuroleptics or benzodiazepines may be needed. Symptoms may subside even without medication. Recurrent episodes of postictal psychosis may evolve into interictal psychosis.

The pathophysiology of psychosis in epilepsy is not known. Bilateral epileptic foci may be more common in patients who develop postictal psychosis. Increased release of dopamine after seizures may play a role. Vigabatrin (VGB), an investigational antiepileptic drug, can induce interictal psychosis. Vigabatrin selectively and irreversibly inhibits gamma-aminobutyric acid (GABA) transaminase, resulting in increased GABA levels, which suggests that alterations in GABA regulation may play a role in psychosis.

Patients with postictal psychosis may present with stereotypical symptoms. After experiencing several seizures in the epilepsy monitoring unit, one patient of mine became obsessed with issues about money. It was virtually the only topic he could speak about for several days, and not in a very rational fashion. Once or twice a year, when he had a flurry of seizures, he developed the same psychotic preoccupation with money.

73. Does Donna have an "epileptic personality?"

Yes.

Debate continues on the very existence of an "epileptic personality." The constellation of hypergraphia, hyposexuality, and hyperreligiosity described in temporal lobe patients is known as the Geschwind syndrome. Additional characteristics that seem overrepresented in patients with temporal lobe epilepsy are emotionality, manic tendencies, depression, humorlessness, altered sexuality, anger, hostility, aggression, religiosity, nascent philosophical interest, augmented sense of personal destiny, dependence, passivity, paranoia, moralism, guilt, obsessionalism, circumstantiality, viscosity, and hypergraphia. It has been hypothesized that the abnormal electrical activity in the limbic system disrupts the regulation of motivation and affect, resulting in this symptom complex.

If we look at Donna's clinical profile, we see that she possesses many of these characteristics. To assess her fairly, she would have to be evaluated in more depth and on more than one visit. However, Donna is overemotional, depressed, without any apparent sense of humor, angry and hostile toward her sister and me, and appears excessively religious, mildly paranoid, circumstantial, and viscous. Some of these symptoms, such as emotionality and depression, could be associated with any illness, and many patients are overly circumstantial. Still, if there is an "epileptic personality," it looks like Donna has it.

In my practice, the most impressive feature of the epileptic personality is viscosity, or "stickiness." These patients do everything they can to prolong the doctor visit and, even after having left the examining room, typically will ask to come back for "just one more question." Clearly, this type of behavior can disrupt a busy office, but it is more comprehensible when seen in the context of the epileptic personality. Circumstantiality and viscosity are notoriously difficult to treat.

74. Was it wise to keep her sister in the room?

Yes.

Patients with epilepsy may suffer from overprotective family members and believe that they are not left to cope independently. On the other hand, many patients lack sufficient insight to know when they need assistance.

I welcome family members on a first visit. They usually provide additional history and a description of the seizures. Family members often have to take time off from work to come to the doctor and may not appear at every visit. They also can serve as witnesses to the examination and explanations given during the visit, which the patient may not accurately recall. There is always the option of seeing the patient alone for a few minutes toward the end of the visit to provide for discussion of confidential matters.

Seeing how Donna treated her sister told me a lot about her level of frustration with her epilepsy, as well as her distressed mood and need for continued psychiatric care. Social work intervention can also assist many patients with epilepsy regarding location of services such as transportation, free medication, and support groups. The social worker also may identify and address caretaker needs.

75. Can control of the epilepsy worsen behavioral symptoms?

Yes.

The theory of "forced normalization" is another controversial topic. Originally applied to the observation that electroencephalogram (EEG) abnormalities could normalize when the patient became psychotic, the concept has been extended to clinical behavior. Some patients appear to have worsening of their psychosis or depression when seizures improve. The recurrence of seizures may terminate the psychosis. Other symptoms, such as angry outbursts, agitation, mania, and anxiety states, may also increase in the face of decreased seizure frequency.

This phenomenon is particularly striking after successful epilepsy surgery, when depression may worsen or psychosis present for the first time. One of my patients, who had always been able to manage her depression as an outpatient, required psychiatric hospitalization several months after a right temporal lobectomy had eliminated the vast majority of her seizures.

How much of the inverse relationship between seizures and behavioral abnormalities relates to elements of psychosocial adjustment versus physiologic factors affecting limbic structures remains speculative.

76. What is the worst thing about living with epilepsy?

Fear of another seizure.

Although seizures take up only minutes in the lives of most patients during the year, the threat of a seizure at any time can create a chronic disabling condition. In one study, almost half the respondents volunteered that fear of another seizure troubled them the most. Many worry about the possibility of injury during a seizure (see Chapter 9).

A large number of patients with uncontrolled epilepsy find that the inability to drive is a major stress and limiting factor in their lives. Some states require mandatory reporting of patients with epilepsy (see Resource Y). If not handled properly, the issue of driving may create a rift in the patient-doctor relationship.

Unemployment of people with epilepsy is double the rate of the general population. Lack of employment can lead to difficulty obtaining health insurance. Other concerns are problems at work and social stigma.

Marriage rates are lower for people with epilepsy, particularly men. Divorce rates are similar to those of the rest of the population.

Although neurologists spend most of their energy addressing seizure classification and frequency, it is clear that epilepsy is a disorder that has a significant impact on a patient's psychosocial well-being. The resources of a social worker, neuropsychologist, and psychiatrist can often help clarify and alleviate symptoms of depression, suicidal ideation, and psychosis.

8

Epilepsy in the Elderly

Unhappy with the diagnosis of epilepsy made by two other neurologists, Joan came to me for a second opinion. Now 73 years old, she complains of "sick feelings" for the last 25 years. These "paranoid or sinking-like feelings" last three to five seconds, occur three to four times a month, and began just after her menopause. They are never associated with palpitations, shortness of breath, diaphoresis, alteration of consciousness, lip smacking, picking movements, or with olfactory, auditory, or visual hallucinations. Although she had described these events to her doctors over the years, no one ever came up with a diagnosis. She feels uneasy and fearful during the spells. She insisted that no one other than herself could tell that she was having a spell.

That contention changed abruptly six months ago. Joan had another one of her typical "sick feelings," then became stiff and fell backward. There was no tongue biting or incontinence. She claims that she was not confused, but this is disputed by her daughter, who witnessed her crash to the floor and make some jerking movements. Her mother lay there for several minutes before getting up.

Joan's past medical history was remarkable for decreased hearing bilaterally with a left cochlear implant. Because of her poor hearing, she cannot talk on the phone or keep up with her friends. She has become depressed and attributes this condition to her social isolation. She had been in a motor vehicle accident 20 years before the onset of her spells, and her head struck the windshield. She thinks she was unconscious for a few minutes.

A cardiac evaluation for syncope resulted in a normal physical examination, electrocardiogram, Holter monitor, and echocardiogram.

*A computed axial tomography (CAT) scan was of limited value
because of extensive artifact caused by her cochlear implant. Her first
electroencephalogram (EEG) revealed bilateral sharp waves in the temporal regions. A repeat EEG was normal. She cannot have a magnetic
resonance imaging scan because of the cochlear implant.*

*Her first neurologist told her that the feelings she had been experi-
encing were classic epileptic auras and that she had a seizure disorder.
He prescribed phenytoin, 300 mg at night. Joan found that when she
got up in the morning, she was unable to walk straight. Worried that
she might fall and break her hip like her sister, she immediately
stopped taking the medication without consulting the doctor.*

*Four months later, on no medication except her fluoxetine (Prozac),
she has had no more spells, feels great, but wonders if she should be
driving because of her epilepsy. She has had no more abnormal feelings or any type of spell.*

*When I examined her, I found a mild bilateral intention tremor. She
made a slight mistake recalling the date and after five minutes could
remember only two words of three. Her partial deafness made commu-
nicating with her challenging and significantly increased the duration
of the interview and examination.*

Questions

77. Does Joan have epilepsy?

I couldn't be sure.

The incidence of epilepsy is high during infancy, decreases in childhood and adolescence, remains stable in middle age, and increases
again in the elderly. The risk of developing epilepsy rises from 1 percent
at age 20 to 3 percent at age 75. Consequently, it would be a bit unusual for this patient to develop epilepsy in her late forties. Stroke and
tumor are the two most common causes of seizures in the older population, and Joan has evidence of neither. Of course, her CAT scan was of
such poor resolution that she could have a small brain tumor in her temporal lobe, perhaps a low-grade glioma. But without a magnetic resonance imaging scan, there would be no easy way to make the diagnosis.

One could explain her 25 years of "paranoid feelings" as partial simple seizures. She denied alteration of consciousness, but did volunteer
that she was afraid when she had these feelings and did not want to be
alone. The larger spell she had would be classified as a partial seizure
with secondary generalization. Of course, the small spells might also
represent panic attacks related to anxiety, and it may just have been

coincidence that she had a syncopal event right after one of those feelings. It may also be that her fall represents her first epileptic convulsion and may not be related to the feelings of panic. Even a detailed history with a witness does not always provide sufficient information to make a definite diagnosis.

The incidence of epilepsy in the elderly is greater than in any other age group. Each year in the United States, more than 41,000 elderly suffer their first symptomatic seizure. Seizures usually can be controlled with one antiepileptic drug (AED).

78. Is the head injury related?

The risk of developing epilepsy after a closed head injury ranges from 3 percent to 7 percent.

Factors that increase the risk of developing seizures are prolonged unconsciousness or posttraumatic amnesia (greater than 24 hours), brain contusion, or intracerebral hematoma. Most patients who are going to develop epilepsy from a head injury do so within five years. There is no detectable increase in risk for individuals with mild head injury (amnesia or loss of consciousness of less than one half hour's duration). Given that the head injury occurred 20 years before the onset of Joan's spells and because she has none of the risk factors associated with a severe head injury, it is unlikely that her concussion played a role in the etiology of these spells.

79. Does she need an antiepileptic drug?

No.

Her spells have disappeared for the moment. I told her that as long as her diagnosis is not certain, she could stay off antiepileptic medication for now. On the other hand, should her spells return, I would like to study her a bit more. Ideally, we should try to capture one of these spells with EEG monitoring, either as an inpatient with video-EEG telemetry or as an outpatient with a home monitoring system. If these studies show epileptic activity during the spell, we have an answer. However, the diagnosis would still be in doubt if they do not, given the fact that scalp electrodes do not always record partial simple seizures. In that case, it would be reasonable to try a low dose of another AED, such as carbamazepine. Phenytoin and carbamazepine are the drugs of choice for the treatment of partial seizures. (Gabapentin is another AED that plays a particular role in seizure control in the elderly by virtue of its lack of drug interactions.)

Carbamazepine is now available in two slow-release forms that have the advantage of more constant drug levels and lower incidence of toxic side effects. One of these is Tegretol XR; the other is Carbatrol (see Resource I). I would begin with a very low dose, such as 100 mg twice a day, and titrate to response or side effects, whichever came first. Another option would be phenytoin 100 mg at bedtime. If Joan tolerates it, she could increase to 100 mg twice a day to get her serum level into the therapeutic range.

80. Was the 300 mg dose of phenytoin too high for her?

Yes.

Although many adults tolerate a 300 mg bedtime dose of phenytoin, the elderly are more susceptible to AED side effects and require lower doses. Multiple factors increase the sensitivity of the elderly to medications. Aging results in decreased hepatic enzyme activity and hepatic blood flow. In addition, glomerular filtration rate, tubular secretory function, and renal blood flow also decrease. Hepatic drug metabolism and renal function drop 10 percent per year after age 40.

The results of these physiologic changes are longer elimination half-life and decreased drug clearance. In patients aged 60 to 79 years, phenytoin metabolism is reduced by approximately 20 percent. Similarly, because gabapentin is renally cleared, doses need to be reduced 30 percent to 50 percent in the elderly. The elimination half-life of diazepam increases from 15 hours for an 18-year-old to 100 hours for a healthy 95-year-old. Doses must be adjusted accordingly.

Because many elderly patients have hypoalbuminemia, the free active fraction of the AED is increased, which leads to increased side effects and increased therapeutic effects at a given dose.

Like many patients who experience AED side effects, Joan stopped the medication without informing her physician. This turn of events left her unprotected from another possible seizure and undermined her doctor-patient relationship.

81. Could there be an adverse interaction between phenytoin and fluoxetine?

Yes.

Drug interactions occur more often than not in the elderly. The most frequent type of drug interaction occurs due to changes in hepatic metabolism. Drug toxicity represents a major medical problem in the geriatric population. Two thirds of patients over the age of 60 take prescription medications, and more than half of the elderly take more than three medications. Patients in chronic care facilities who take AEDs often receive at least five other medications. Joan is a little unusual in that she needs only one other medication.

However, fluoxetine is a selective serotonin reuptake inhibitor (SSRI), a class of medication that inhibits the cytochrome P450 system. Fluoxetine has been reported to increase both phenytoin and carbamazepine levels, producing anticonvulsant toxicity. This effect may have contributed to Joan's phenytoin intolerance.

Phenytoin levels also may be increased by the tricyclic antidepressant imipramine. Should Joan require an AED in the future, one that does not pass through the cytochrome P450 system would not cause these drug interactions. Gabapentin undergoes no hepatic metabolism.

82. Would carbamazepine be a good treatment if Joan has a second seizure?

Yes.

Like phenytoin, carbamazepine levels can be increased by fluoxetine. Consequently, a low dose of carbamazepine should be used at the onset and drug levels should be closely followed.

Carbamazepine-induced hyponatremia occurs more frequently in the elderly. Hypertension and diuretic use are other risk factors. Inappropriate release of antidiuretic hormone and a renal tubular effect appear responsible. Hemodilution or insufficient salt intake may aggravate the condition. Carbamazepine-induced hyponatremia only occasionally produces symptoms. Convulsions usually do not occur until the serum sodium is less than 115 mEq/L, or sometimes at a higher level if the sodium drops rapidly.

The Carbatrol slow-release preparation is composed of sprinkles, which can be mixed with soft food for patients who have trouble swallowing capsules. Bioavailability does not change. (The Tegretol XR tablet cannot be broken and still work properly.)

In patients with underlying cardiac conduction defects, carbamazepine can induce arrhythmias such as sinus arrest, bundle branch block, fascicular block, sinus bradycardia and bradycardia-tachycardia syndrome. The incidence of these arrhythmias is not known. A baseline electrocardiogram before initiation of carbamazepine therapy is prudent.

Despite these caveats, carbamazepine may be a very useful drug in the elderly. The choice of AED therapy must be individualized. There currently are no results from controlled trials in the elderly to rely on for guidance in prescribing AEDs.

83. If Joan has epilepsy, is it likely to show on the electroencephalo-gram?

No.

As mentioned in question 79, partial simple seizures often are not visible on the scalp EEG. Consequently, even if one of Joan's attacks of fear were recorded, the EEG result could be a false-negative. Partial seizures are the most common type of seizure to present in patients over 60 years old. These often are associated with a focal lesion such as a stroke or tumor.

In addition, the interictal EEG is less likely to show epileptic activity in the elderly. In patients with a mean age of 70 whose seizure onset occurred after 60 years of age, only 26 percent of initial EEGs demonstrated epileptiform activity. In contrast, the yield of a first EEG may be as high as 77 percent in children. Older patients with a seizure frequency of at least one seizure per month were more likely to have positive EEGs.

Prolonged EEG recording can be useful if the initial EEG is normal, but epilepsy is still suspected. Inpatient video-EEG or outpatient ambulatory monitoring yield far more data than a 20-minute routine EEG and increase the likelihood of a positive study. Repeating a routine EEG with sleep deprivation also can yield better results if an initial study is negative.

Joan's EEGs gave conflicting results. One suggested a nonspecific disturbance bilaterally, whereas the second was normal. Mild temporal slowing can be normal in the elderly. Joan's EEG also may have been distorted by the skull defect in the left temporal region related to her cochlear implant. A transient metabolic disturbance may have been responsible for the first abnormal EEG. The nonspecific findings might result from her concussion at the time of her motor vehicle accident. No definitive diagnosis of epilepsy can be made from the available information.

84. Is it a coincidence that Joan's seizures began just after her menopause?

Probably not.

Pituitary gonadotropins increase at menopause, whereas estrogen and progesterone decrease. Seizure worsening has been reported after menopause, and some women find that hormone replacement therapy changes seizure patterns. In patients who have catamenial seizures, the cyclic pattern of their seizures disappears with menopause. First seizures may also occur with menopause.

85. Should Joan be driving?

Yes.

The driving issue is always a sensitive one. Technically, Joan does not have epilepsy, which is a condition of recurrent seizures. At least I could not make the diagnosis by history, examination, or with the aid of two EEGs. She has been "spell-free" for four months. If her small spells for the last 25 years were epileptic seizures, they did not impair her consciousness or her driving. The single larger spell is still a mystery. Since she has been off medications and spell-free, it seems reasonable to let her continue to drive. She already suffers from depression, at least partially related to decreased social interaction resulting from her impaired hearing. Not being able to drive would isolate her further.

If it were definite that Joan had epilepsy, most states would not permit her to drive until she was seizure-free for a longer period of time, such as six or 12 months. However, for a number of states, three months seizure-free is sufficient (see Resource Y).

Joan should be followed up closely so that any new symptoms can be investigated. A repeat EEG may be fruitful in the future.

9

Seizures and Alcohol

A 58-year-old white man with a history of chronic alcohol abuse woke his wife at 3:30 a.m. with a loud cry. George was sweaty, weak, and incontinent of urine. His wife ran to the next room to call an ambulance. When she returned, his body was stiff and he drooled bloody saliva. George had a witnessed generalized tonic-clonic seizure in the ambulance. He had another convulsion upon arrival at the emergency room (ER). He received diazepam, lorazepam, meperidine, intravenous glucose, and potassium.

George's medical history was notable for mild hypertension and multiple failed attempts at detoxification. After years of enduring his alcoholism, his wife threatened to leave last week. George takes metoprolol, premarin, hydrochlorothiazide, and vitamins. He has no allergies. He smokes one pack of cigarettes per day.

Although he was very groggy in the ER, George mumbled that his last drink was two weeks ago, when he went on a binge and guzzled three bottles of wine. He does not use illicit drugs. He has no history of head injury or delirium tremens. Alcoholism is his only risk factor for seizures.

Examination revealed him to be afebrile with a heart rate of 120/minute. Blood pressure was 170/100 and respirations were 24/minute. His disheveled gray hair, sallow complexion, and wrinkled face made him appear older than his stated age. He knew it was a Sunday in September, but he could not state the date. He answered slowly and his words were slurred. He could follow simple but not complex commands.

An examination limited by pain suggested a dislocated shoulder. Physical and neurologic examinations were otherwise normal. The ER physician put George's right upper extremity in a sling.

Laboratory values: Na 129 meq/l, CO2 20 meq/l, Cl 91 meq/l, K 2.1 meq/l, BUN 22 mg/dl, creatinine 1.3 mg/dl, glucose 110 mg/dl, AST 46 Karmen units, PT and PTT normal. White count 22,500/cubic millimeter, hemoglobin 13.1 g/dl, platelets 267,000/cubic millimeter. Alcohol level, drug screen, and urinalysis were negative. EKG revealed sinus tachycardia. Computerized axial tomography (CAT) scan of the brain showed mild atrophy. An electroencephalogram (EEG) and magnetic resonance imaging (MRI) scan were ordered.

Questions

86. Were George's seizures caused by alcoholism?

Probably.

Patients with seizures related to alcohol can best be divided into three groups:

- Patients with chronic alcoholism who have withdrawal seizures
- Patients with idiopathic epilepsy in whom alcohol exacerbates their seizures
- Patients with alcoholism and associated cerebral trauma

More than 75 percent of patients with alcoholic withdrawal seizures have them within 7 to 30 hours after alcohol cessation. However, a few patients have seizures within hours after the last drink, or seizures may occur as long as 5 to 20 days later.

My patient's seizures occurred two weeks after his last drink, which suggests that there may be another etiology besides alcohol withdrawal. However, 14 days is still within the 20-day time period reported by Maurice Victor. (Determining the number of days since the last drink is problematic if the patient is the only one providing the information.) George is tachycardic, which may be a sign of alcohol withdrawal. Alternative explanations of his rapid heart rate include seizures, shoulder pain, and the stress of the late-night ER visit.

Delirium tremens (DTs), a syndrome that is characterized by tremor, agitation, sensory hallucinations, and increased autonomic nervous system activity, typically occurs 72 to 96 hours after the cessation of drinking. When seizures and DTs occur, seizures occur first. George does not appear to have the DTs, at least not yet. Hospital admission is mandatory given the cluster of seizures and the potential for DTs. Five percent of hospitalized alcoholics develop DTs. Mortality from DTs is approximately 10 percent.

Because as many as 7 percent of alcoholics have convulsive seizures, alcohol seems the most likely etiology for new-onset seizures in this patient. The incidence of seizures increases with the severity of the alcoholism.

87. If alcohol withdrawal didn't cause his seizures, what did?

Multiple possibilities require thorough diagnostic evaluation and hospitalization.

Other causes of seizures in this population include metabolic (hypocalcemia, hypoglycemia, hyponatremia, hypomagnesemia, uremia, hepatic encephalopathy), toxic ingestion, meningitis, encephalitis, cerebral abscess, brain contusion, subdural or intracerebral hematoma, subarachnoid hemorrhage, stroke, and neoplasm.

George's serum sodium is low at 129 meq/l. Hyponatremia can cause seizures, particularly when the serum sodium drops below 115 meq/l. If the serum sodium falls rapidly, levels as high as 125 to 130 meq/l can result in confusion and lethargy. Seizures could occur at a serum sodium level of 129 meq/l. However, this mild hyponatremia is most likely the result of the patient's diuretic treatment for hypertension. The hydrochlorothiazide is probably also responsible for his low serum potassium.

Alcohol is one of the most common drugs that causes hypoglycemia. Because hypoglycemia can cause seizures, any patient with new-onset seizures must have a serum glucose checked. George's serum glucose was normal. On presentation to the ER, he also received intravenous glucose as an emergency measure. It is important to remember to administer thiamine (50–100 mg) intravenously before the glucose infusion to avoid precipitating the ataxia, confusion, and ophthalmoplegia of Wernicke's syndrome.

When severe (<0.8 meq/l), hypomagnesemia can be associated with seizures. Hypophosphatemia may occur with alcohol withdrawal and can cause generalized tonic clonic seizures at phosphate levels less than 1 mg/dl. Both magnesium and phosphate levels should be checked.

Of course, the patient needs a drug screen to eliminate possible causes of seizures such as cocaine, amphetamines, phencyclidine, or heroin. Substance abuse is often associated with alcohol abuse. The patient also may have withdrawal seizures from a prescription of sedatives that has run out, such as benzodiazepines or barbiturates. Benzodiazepines are prescribed for 1.5 percent of Americans, often to control anxiety and promote sleep. It would not be surprising if

George had obtained a prescription for benzodiazepines to help with his withdrawal symptoms and depression about his pending marriage breakup.

It also is possible that George has an underlying cause for epilepsy that has been unmasked by the alcohol. A subtle brain lesion such as a heterotopia or gyral malformation might be seen on an MRI, but not on a CAT scan. He may have mesial temporal sclerosis, which typically is not seen on a CAT scan. A silent stroke, such as an ischemic infarct in the occipital lobe, could be epileptogenic. Strokes and brain trauma occur more frequently in alcoholics.

The discovery of such an underlying cause for his seizures would help prognostically, as the seizures are more likely to recur. The presence of a fixed lesion also would favor treatment with antiepileptic medication.

88. Why is George confused?

He probably is postictal.

The causes of encephalopathy are legion, including metabolic, toxic, neoplastic, infectious, endocrine, structural, and other abnormalities. As mentioned previously, hyponatremia, if acute, could be responsible. Another possibility is a central nervous system infection (see question 89).

George awoke with arm pain, probably having dislocated his shoulder as a result of a convulsion in his sleep. His wife then witnessed him becoming stiff and drooling as he had a tonic seizure. Blood from his mouth indicated that he had bitten his tongue. He then had two more brief convulsions. Four generalized seizures typically produce a postictal state of lethargy and confusion that lasts from minutes to hours. The corresponding finding in his EEG most likely would be generalized slowing.

A focal deficit after a seizure, a Todd's paralysis, can point to the anatomic focus of the seizure. Todd's paralysis typically lasts a few minutes but may last as long as two days. George's neurologic examination did not provide any evidence of a Todd's paralysis.

Lorazepam and diazepam were administered in the ER to control his seizures. George also received meperidine for shoulder pain. All three of these medications contribute to his altered mental status.

Another possibility for his lack of return to normal mental status is nonconvulsive status epilepticus (see question 90).

89. Does George need a lumbar puncture?

Yes.

A lumbar puncture (LP) should be performed whenever one suspects central nervous system (CNS) infection. Alcoholic patients are at increased risk for meningitis. Meningitis and encephalitis can be successfully treated, but antibiotics must be started promptly.

A less common indication for LP is suspicion of occult intracerebral hemorrhage as a result of a leaky aneurysm. Because both CNS infection and hemorrhage can precipitate seizures, an LP is often helpful in a first seizure.

George had been well until he went to bed. In the ER he was mildly confused but not agitated, and without fever. He did not have a stiff neck. Meningitis seemed an unlikely diagnosis.

On the other hand, he had never had seizures and now presents with four in a row. There was no definite history of alcohol withdrawal. He remains mildly confused, is tachycardic, and has an elevated white count. His white count elevation may be due to the stress of the seizures or may represent an underlying infection. The CAT scan did not show an infarct, hemorrhage, or subdural hematoma to explain his seizures. Although there is no strong evidence of meningitis, the lack of another probable etiology (other than alcoholism) warrants an LP.

90. Does George need an electroencephalogram?

Yes, but not right now.

In the ER, the main purpose of an EEG is to see whether the patient is still seizing. Short of that, the EEG may reveal focal abnormalities (spikes or slow waves), pointing to a seizure focus or underlying brain lesion such as a tumor or stroke. In this patient, the normal CAT scan reassures us that no large structural lesion is responsible for his seizures. (An acute stroke may have been missed by the CAT scan and should be detected by MRI.)

Although the patient is no longer having convulsions, one must consider whether his confusion is due to continued seizures that are not clinically obvious. These may be detected on examination by eye fluttering or intermittent twitching of a hand or the face. Continued subclinical seizures can damage the CNS. If there is any question regarding the possibility of subclinical seizures, order a stat EEG to look for continuing electrographic epileptic activity.

If George is postictal, he should progressively become more alert. He requires close observation with frequent neurologic checkup by the nursing staff. Because George woke up and continued to improve clinically, the EEG was performed the next day. It showed mild generalized slowing consistent with encephalopathy and superimposed fast activity related to benzodiazepine treatment. There was no photomyoclonus or photoconvulsive response. (Photomyoclonus or photoconvulsions induced by the strobe light occur in approximately one half of patients in the throes of alcohol withdrawal. When they are not in withdrawal, these patients typically have normal EEGs (see Resource Z).

91. Should I start daily anticonvulsant medication?

Yes.

George had three witnessed seizures. He probably had a fourth, which dislocated his shoulder and startled his wife. George did not fully return to consciousness during his flurry of seizures, and consequently had status epilepticus (SE) (see Chapter 10). At this point, with the etiology of the seizures still not known, and the high mortality that accompanies SE, there really is no choice but to begin antiepileptic drug (AED) therapy.

Alcohol may be responsible for as many as 25 percent of cases of SE. If the seizures are due to alcohol withdrawal, they may well be self-limited and not require maintenance AED therapy. Ninety percent of patients with alcohol withdrawal seizures have fewer than six seizures. Most seizures in alcoholic patients are due to alcohol withdrawal.

Because the patient is not seizing now, at least as far as we can tell (see question 90 regarding subclinical seizures), he does not need additional intravenous (IV) diazepam or lorazepam. The most commonly used IV medications for chronic treatment of seizures are phenobarbital and phenytoin. I would choose the latter because he is already confused and is likely to become more sedated from phenobarbital.

Valproic acid is now available in an IV form (Depakon), but it has no clear advantages over phenytoin in this setting and is not yet indicated for the treatment of SE. Intravenous phenytoin is now available as fosphenytoin (Cerebyx), a water-soluble phenytoin prodrug. Although it is more expensive than phenytoin, fosphenytoin causes less discomfort at the injection site. Cardiovascular complications may also be reduced. I loaded George with phenytoin at 15 mg/kg and began a maintenance dose of 100 mg intravenously three times a day. I followed phenytoin levels daily during his hospitalization. He had no further seizures in hospital.

If George's seizures are related to alcoholism, he probably will not require ongoing therapy with an oral AED once he leaves the hospital. The likelihood that he will be compliant enough to benefit from the medication is low. If he does take phenytoin and continues to drink, he will need higher doses of phenytoin to achieve therapeutic levels because of increased phenytoin clearance related to the effect of chronic ethanol on the hepatic microsomal enzyme system. The usefulness of phenytoin in seizure control in this setting remains in doubt. Abstinence is the best prophylaxis for alcohol-related seizures.

92. George dislocated his shoulder. Are injuries common with epileptic seizures?

Yes.

Five percent of patients with epilepsy visit the ER each year because of a seizure-induced injury. Head injuries are the most common. In one study, 24 percent of patients had a head injury the previous year. Most head injuries are mild, but they may be severe, including skull fracture or intracranial clot. Many require sutures.

Patients with convulsions, more than one seizure per month, and adverse effects from their AEDs are all more likely to have injuries. Patients with atonic seizures are at high risk for injury.

As many as 15 percent of patients with convulsions sustain vertebral compression fractures. These are typically thoracic between T3 and T8 and usually are asymptomatic. They occur more frequently in the elderly and during nocturnal seizures. Fractures of the shoulder, humerus, and hip also may occur. One patient has been reported with simultaneous central dislocation of a hip with fracture of the contralateral femoral neck.

Shoulder dislocations, like George's, may be anterior or posterior. They may recur with repeated seizures. The extreme muscle contraction during the convulsion causes the injury.

Burns typically occur at home. In one report, 40 percent of burns were due to cooking and 20 percent occurred in the shower. Skin grafting may be necessary. The risk of burns can be lessened by using a microwave oven for cooking, eliminating exposed room heaters, and minimizing the use of hot objects such as electric burners and curling irons (see Resource T).

The most common cause of accidental death due to a seizure is drowning. Patients at risk should not swim alone or even use whirlpools or bathtubs without supervision. Fishing and falling into water may result in drowning.

93. Why did George receive both lorazepam and diazepam?

There is no known clinical advantage for mixing the two.

Lorazepam or diazepam can control acute seizures. These benzodiazepines also diminish symptoms of alcohol withdrawal. There is no clear superiority between lorazepam and diazepam for seizure control (see discussion in Chapter 10, question 104.) Diazepam enters the brain more rapidly, but lorazepam lasts longer.

Intravenous rate of administration of lorazepam or diazepam should not exceed 2 mg/minute. Lorazepam can be given intramuscularly if necessary. Both drugs are effective for SE. Heavy smokers require higher doses of benzodiazepines because of nicotine-induced hepatic microsomal enzymes. Patients with liver failure have impaired drug clearance and should receive lower doses. Lorazepam is more expensive.

In order to better predict medication effect, choose one drug or the other in a given patient.

94. Will mild drinking increase seizure frequency in people with epilepsy?

Rarely.

Alcohol abuse can induce seizures, but there is no evidence that light drinking exacerbates seizure disorders. This may seem surprising given the tradition of advising epileptic patients to refrain from drinking. A study of 5,000 adolescent patients with epilepsy found that moderate drinking did not increase their seizure frequency. One careful study of hospitalized epileptic inpatients who were given controlled amounts of alcohol on a regular basis failed to reveal any increase in their seizures.

Another study looked at the EEG in patients with epilepsy and failed to detect activation of epileptic abnormalities by alcohol. In fact, alcohol caused a transient suppression of epileptic activity. A "rebound" phenomenon occurred in a few patients, in whom the epileptic activity increased above baseline 12 to 24 hours later.

There is no clinical information to bolster a blanket recommendation that patients with seizures refrain from all alcohol consumption. Heavy drinking can exacerbate seizures. Excessive alcohol use may also be associated with sleep deprivation, stress, and missed medication doses, which contribute to breakthrough seizures. Heavy regular alcohol consumption and binge drinking increase seizure frequency.

Whether alcohol intake adversely affects a patient's overall health is a different question. A patient's alcohol consumption should be evaluated in the clinical context of his medical history and social milieu.

95. In patients with epilepsy, how does alcohol ingestion affect their antiepileptic drugs?

It depends.

One must first distinguish between acute and chronic alcohol ingestion. Acutely, alcohol can compete with the metabolism of AEDs and prolong their half-lives. For example, barbiturate elimination is slowed during alcoholic intoxication. This phenomenon can lead to toxicity and death from the combination of the two drugs.

Chronic alcohol use hypertrophies smooth endoplasmic reticulum and induces cytochrome P450 enzymes. Consequently, AEDs such as carbamazepine, phenobarbital, phenytoin, and primidone undergo more efficient metabolism. Patients will need larger doses of these drugs to maintain therapeutic serum levels. Multiple daily doses of AEDs also provide more constant serum levels.

Chronic alcoholics may have cirrhosis with hypoalbuminemia. The low albumin results in higher free levels of normally tightly bound drugs such as carbamazepine, phenytoin, and valproate. These free levels can have greater toxic as well as therapeutic effect. Acetaldehyde, a metabolite of ethanol, can also compete with AEDs for albumin-binding sites, increasing free AED levels. Patients with significant hypoalbuminemia or ethanol intake who are difficult to manage may benefit from measurement of free AED levels.

10

Generalized Convulsive Status Epilepticus

Laura was a healthy 11-year-old girl who hit a pothole with her skateboard, fell to the ground, and struck her head. According to her girlfriend, Laura cried out and began to shake all over. She drooled and turned blue. Laura was still convulsing when the ambulance arrived. Despite 10 mg of intravenous (IV) diazepam and a loading dose of fosphenytoin, her seizures continued in the emergency room (ER).

Laura's birth and development were normal. She never had a head injury, meningitis, encephalitis, or a febrile seizure. Although no one in her family had epilepsy, her brother experienced two simple febrile seizures when he was three years old.

A good student, Laura had no behavioral problems. She didn't use alcohol or drugs. She had just begun her first menstrual period three days before the accident.

In the ER, she received a total of 20 mg of diazepam and 1,000 mg of phenytoin equivalents of fosphenytoin. Because her respirations were shallow, the ER physician intubated her and connected her to a ventilator. He breathed a sigh of relief when the convulsions finally stopped after 45 minutes. He sent her for a computed axial tomography (CAT) scan, which was normal.

The neurologist examined Laura after she returned from the radiology department. Her temperature was 101.2°F. Her head was atraumatic, without facial bruising or blood behind her tympanic membranes. Pupils were equal and reactive, fundi normal, neck supple, tone normal, and reflexes equal. She did not have any Babinski signs.

Electrolytes and chemistry panels were normal. Her white blood cell count was elevated to 17,000/cubic mm with only a few bands. A urine dipstick was normal. An arterial blood gas from admission revealed a pH of 7.10, a pCO_2 of 55 mmHg, and an O_2 of 70 mmHg.

As the neurologist packed up his black bag, he noticed Laura's left cheek twitch. He pulled the covers down and saw Laura's left hand jerk slightly. He called the electroencephalograph (EEG) technician at home to arrange for a stat EEG. He ordered 10 mg more of diazepam and a phenytoin level.

An hour later, when the EEG was hooked up, the neurologist saw continuous spike wave activity. He ordered a gram of phenobarbital IV. Then he performed a lumbar puncture to check for meningoencephalitis.

The EEG pattern remained unchanged 30 minutes later. The neurologist transferred Laura to the intensive care unit and started a pentobarbital drip. The EEG electrodes were removed for her to have a magnetic resonance imaging (MRI) scan. After the MRI, which was normal, the technician reattached the electrodes securely with collodion for continuous EEG monitoring throughout the night.

Two hours later, the EEG revealed a burst suppression pattern, with bursts of sharp waves and spikes lasting 1 to 2 seconds separated by periods of suppression lasting 10 to 12 seconds. The lumbar puncture results came back showing five white cells, no red cells, and normal glucose and protein. The neurologist ordered phenytoin and phenobarbital levels for the morning and went to talk to Laura's parents.

Questions

96. Did Laura have status epilepticus?

Yes.

Status epilepticus (SE) is defined as recurrent seizures that are "so frequently repeated or so prolonged as to create a fixed and lasting condition". Status epilepticus occurs in 50,000 to 100,000 people in the United States each year. Approximately half of them are children.

The modern definition of SE includes not only convulsive epilepsy, but also all seizure types, and refers to the persistence or rapid recurrence of seizures. Thirty minutes of epileptic activity is often used as the duration of seizures that qualifies for SE. However, any seizure that lasts longer than a few minutes is out of the ordinary and presents the risk of SE. More than three seizures within 24 hours also warrants aggressive treatment.

97. Could Laura's fever and elevated white count be related to status epilepticus?

Yes.

Status epilepticus commonly produces hyperpyrexia. The physical work of convulsive status, as well as central mechanisms, can elevate body temperature.

Demarginalization secondary to circulating catecholamines during SE can raise the peripheral white count to over 20,000/cubic millimeter. (Bands on the peripheral smear suggest infection.)

Although an elevated fever and white blood cell count do not necessarily point to an infection, patients in SE should be aggressively evaluated for a source of fever. By promptly performing a lumbar puncture, the neurologist eliminated any question that Laura might have meningitis.

98. Are Laura's seizures caused by head trauma?

No.

There was no significant bruising on her scalp, and her CAT scan and MRI were normal. Risk factors for epilepsy after closed head injury include intracranial hematoma, depressed skull fracture with dural tear, and posttraumatic amnesia lasting longer than 24 hours. Her negative brain scans argue against head injury being responsible for her ongoing seizures. The seizure may even have begun while Laura was on her skateboard, causing her fall rather than resulting from it. Her coma probably is due to the continued epileptic activity in her brain rather than a consequence of her fall.

Children younger than five years old have seizures more commonly than adults do within the first week after trauma. However, these "early" seizures do not necessarily predict the development of epilepsy.

99. Can status epilepticus occur in people who have never had epilepsy?

Yes.

As in Laura's case, SE can be the first sign of neurologic disease. As many as 10 percent of children with epilepsy present with SE. In patients 75 years and older, 35 percent of new-onset seizures present as SE. Mortality is higher in this older age group.

More than 60 percent of cases of SE occur in patients—like Laura—who have never had a seizure. The etiology of almost one third of these remains unexplained.

The major causes of SE are alcohol withdrawal, cerebral trauma, drug toxicity, brain tumors, or congenital malformations. In the case of SE due to antiepileptic drug (AED) withdrawal, reinstituting the drug, even at low doses, can rapidly stop the seizures.

100. If Laura recovers from the status epilepticus, will she develop epilepsy?

Not necessarily.

As far as we know, Laura was neurologically normal before this seizure. Her lumbar puncture, CAT scan, and MRI scan are unremarkable. There appears to be no clear cause for her SE, which places her in the "cryptogenic" group of patients with SE. Surprisingly, SE does not bode a worse prognosis for seizure recurrence than does a single seizure in this patient category.

We need to learn more of Laura's history to determine her risk of developing epilepsy. Did she have any episodes of staring spells as a child that might have been absence seizures? Has she had any myoclonic jerks suggesting a myoclonic epilepsy syndrome? Was she ever incontinent at night, perhaps because of an unwitnessed nocturnal convulsion? Will her EEG give us any clues to an epilepsy syndrome after she recovers from this episode of SE?

Patients with "symptomatic" seizures, where a specific underlying cause can be identified, such as tuberous sclerosis or a congenital brain malformation, demonstrate an increased risk of a second seizure after SE. In addition, these "symptomatic" patients also have an increased risk of another episode of SE.

101. Is Laura likely to have another episode of status epilepticus?

No.

Children who were neurologically normal before their first episode of SE have only a 3 percent chance of recurrent SE. Neurologically impaired children, however, have a recurrence risk of almost 50 percent. Consequently, Laura's risk for another episode of SE appears to be very low.

102. Is it a coincidence that Laura just began menarche?

Probably not.

In 1893 Gowers noted that epilepsy could begin at puberty. Turner seconded this observation in 1907. In 1960 Lennox and Lennox identified a relationship between menarche and first seizure in 25 percent of 387 women whose seizures began between the ages of 8 and 20 years.

Other changes in seizures may occur during puberty, including an increase in seizure frequency or recurrence, alteration of seizure type, and, interestingly, even improved seizure control.

Pituitary gonadotrophins and gonadal steroids increase at puberty. Estrogen activates epileptiform discharges on the electroencephalogram, whereas progesterone can decrease interictal spike frequency. Consequently, it is not surprising that puberty impacts seizure occurrence.

103. Was the twitching of Laura's hand and face a seizure?

Yes.

No one can ignore someone who is actively seizing, and such a patient receives rapid treatment in the ER. Occasionally, a type of "electromechanical dissociation" occurs, in which the patient stops physically convulsing but epileptic activity continues in the brain. The patient may appear postictal, but in fact is actively seizing. This abnormal electrical activity may cause neuronal injury and needs to be controlled. The only way to visualize these abnormal brain waves is with electroencephalography.

Some patients exhibit minor symptoms, such as twitching of the face, trunk, or an extremity after a convulsion, providing a visible clue to this "subtle status epilepticus." Others demonstrate no outward signs.

Any patient who does not awaken promptly after a seizure should have an EEG to determine whether epileptic activity persists. If it does, more effective treatment becomes mandatory.

104. Isn't lorazepam better than diazepam to stop seizures acutely?

No.

Although some neurologists prefer lorazepam, others continue to use diazepam. The anticonvulsant effects of lorazepam last three to four times longer than diazepam because of a higher binding affinity to central nervous system (CNS) benzodiazepine receptor sites. However, because of its high lipid solubility, diazepam penetrates the brain more rapidly and has a slightly faster onset of action.

Diazepam's duration of effect in the brain is less than 30 minutes. If diazepam is used to control SE, another AED, such as phenytoin or phenobarbital, must be added to prevent seizure recurrence. For long-term therapy, a maintenance AED is also required in addition to lorazepam.

Both lorazepam and diazepam cause sedation, which complicates assessment of the patient's mental status. Respiratory depression requiring intubation can occur with either drug. Midazolam is another benzodiazepine that sometimes is used to stop seizures.

105. Isn't a gram of phenobarbital too much?

No.

Assuming that Laura weighs 45 kg, the calculated dose of phenobarbital at 20 mg/kg would be 900 mg. Going by the book, 900 mg would be the preferred dose. Laura has no other medical problems and is likely to tolerate a hefty phenobarbital dose. In this instance, the next major step in seizure control is general anesthesia. As it turned out, even the large dose of phenobarbital was ineffective and she required a pentobarbital drip.

The most common error I see in the treatment of SE is too low a dose of AEDs. Patients continue with seizures for hours or even days with "therapeutic" levels of phenytoin and phenobarbital. When a drug does not work, it needs to be increased to the upper limits or higher of its established "therapeutic range." If it still does not work, a new treatment option needs to be employed as soon as possible.

The morbidity and mortality of SE far outweigh the potential risks of AED toxicity. Neuronal injury, particularly in the hippocampus, occurs after 30 minutes of convulsive SE. Status epilepticus can result in focal neurologic deficits, intellectual deterioration, and persistent epilepsy, as well as multiple medical complications.

The greater the duration of SE, the more likely a poor outcome will result. Status epilepticus lasting longer than 1 hour has 10 times the mortality of shorter episodes. Respiratory failure, hypoxia, and hypotension worsen the prognosis and contribute to brain injury. Mortality ranges from 1 percent to 10 percent, depending on the underlying etiology. When treating SE, it helps to rely on a familiar protocol. Protocols can reduce morbidity and mortality (see Resource S).

106. Is Laura at risk for medical complications from status epilepticus?

Yes.

Medical complications from SE can affect every organ system, increasing both morbidity and mortality. Much progress has been made in managing these complications with modern intensive care.

These systemic complications include:

- Autonomic—failure of cerebral autoregulation resulting in cerebral hypoperfusion, hyperpyrexia, diaphoresis, salivary and tracheobronchial hypersecretion
- Cardiovascular—tachycardia, bradycardia, arrhythmias, labile blood pressure
- CNS—cerebral edema, cerebrospinal fluid pleocytosis
- Hormonal—elevations in prolactin, glucagon, growth hormone, and corticotropin
- Musculoskeletal—rhabdomyolysis resulting in myoglobinuria and renal failure
- Liver—hepatic compromise, disseminated intravascular coagulation
- Metabolic—initial hyperglycemia, then hypoglycemia, respiratory and metabolic acidosis, hypokalemia, hyperkalemia, hyponatremia, hyperazotemia
- Pulmonary—aspiration pneumonia, pulmonary edema from altered lymph flow

In addition, treatment poses iatrogenic risks; benzodiazepines and barbiturates depress respiratory drive, barbiturates cause myocardial depression, and the propylene glycol vehicle in standard phenytoin solution precipitates hypotension and cardiac arrhythmias. Preventing and managing all of these complications constitutes an ongoing challenge for the physician who is taking care of a patient in SE.

107. Will Laura have brain damage from this episode of status epilepticus?

Probably some.

Because of the prolonged epileptic activity—over 30 minutes—Laura is likely to have some neuronal damage, particularly in the hippocampus. However, no cognitive deficits can be demonstrated in many patients with SE and in others, cognitive deficits appear mild.

Most of the morbidity and mortality of SE stem from the etiology of the acute brain insult, such as meningitis, trauma, or stroke. The underlying cause is the most important prognostic factor in convulsive

SE. The prognosis tends to be better when SE occurs because of AED withdrawal or alcohol abuse. Medical complications such as hypotension and sepsis can add to the CNS injury.

Laura has no defined CNS precipitant for her SE, and she is otherwise healthy and likely to be well managed in the intensive care unit, so her risk of significant cognitive sequelae remains low.

108. Are all types of status epilepticus this dangerous?

No.

Absence SE can last days to weeks before diagnosis. Although confused, patients may perform simple tasks of daily living such as getting dressed, eating, and drinking. Absence SE recurs fairly commonly. Seventy-five percent of cases occur in children or adolescents. Absence SE usually is seen in patients with prior seizures, but it may be the presenting symptom of epilepsy.

Carbamazepine treatment of primary generalized epilepsy can cause absence SE. Typical absence seizures do not result in neuronal damage and respond well to IV diazepam or lorazepam.

Confusion is the most common symptom of partial complex SE. Although partial complex SE rarely produces lasting neurologic deficits, some cases have been reported. There remains controversy over how aggressively to treat this type of SE. Most patients with partial complex SE respond to conventional AEDs and do not require anesthetic agents.

11

Nonepileptic Seizures

Kim is a 23-year-old woman whom I met at the epilepsy monitoring unit. She has experienced strange spells for the last four years. Without warning, she becomes weak and her body shakes. Sometimes she feels short of breath and her heart pounds. With more severe episodes, she becomes dizzy and has trouble speaking. Her neurologist sent her to the hospital to see whether we could capture a spell with video and electroencephalographic (EEG) telemetry.

Symptoms began during her freshman year in college. The doctor at student health thought they might be panic attacks and referred Kim to the school psychologist. When the spells continued, a psychiatrist prescribed clonazepam. The medication seemed to help, but she still had attacks once or twice a month. They occurred at any time of day without obvious triggers.

There is no history of problems with gestation, birth, or development. At age 13, Kim fell off the uneven bars during a gymnastics routine and was unconscious for five minutes. She did not have febrile seizures, meningitis, or encephalitis. She never has myoclonic jerks. No auditory, epigastric, olfactory, or visual aura precedes the spells. They are not catamenial. There is no family history of epilepsy.

Kim's parents abruptly divorced when she was 9 years old, but her mother never talks about it. Kim recently has tried to get back in touch with her father, but she has not yet located him.

While in high school, Kim had symptoms of anorexia and bulimia. She told me she "outgrew" the problem. Last year she fell while rollerblading and broke her right wrist. Otherwise she has been well. She takes clonazepam, 1 mg twice a day, and a nonsteroidal antiinflammatory for menstrual cramps. She is allergic to penicillin and sulfa.

Kim smokes two packs of cigarettes a day. She does not abuse drugs or alcohol. Just before graduation she eloped with a new boyfriend. They had not been getting along and separated two weeks ago. Her mother thinks they should get divorced.

Kim majored in psychology and works as a research assistant at the local psychiatric hospital. She has not yet decided whether to go to graduate school and become a counselor.

Last month she had a severe spell at work. She wasn't feeling well anyway and had gone to the doctor the previous day because of a sore throat and muscle aches. He gave her a prescription of antibiotics for the "flu."

Kim said she suddenly felt "funny" and "isolated." She told the secretary, "I am about to have a seizure." She went to her supervisor's office and asked her to help find her doctor's phone number. Her body trembled and she felt as if she would pass out. She tried to dial the phone and couldn't. She felt frustrated and cried. She said "No, no." Then Kim collapsed on the floor and someone said she was having a seizure. There was no tongue biting or incontinence. They told her in the emergency room (ER) that she might be allergic to the antibiotic. Her blood count and chemistries were normal.

Kim told me the story clearly and without obvious distress. She seemed to have good recall of the details.

An ER physician referred her to a neurologist, who said she had an "abnormal" EEG, but a normal magnetic resonance imaging (MRI) scan. He did not recommend antiepileptic drugs.

When I examined Kim, she was cooperative, but a little "giggly." She seemed immature for a married college graduate. Her height was 5 feet 6 inches, and she weighed 120 pounds. Physical and neurologic examinations were normal.

I explained to Kim the purpose of her admission and decreased her clonazepam to 1 mg/day. Early the next morning, she had an episode of heart racing and hand tremors that lasted several minutes. Her EEG was normal. She said it was only a "mild" spell.

The next morning, just after I finished seeing her on rounds, the nurse hurried me back into the room because another spell had started. Kim's hands and trunk trembled, and she seemed very upset. She tried to talk but did not seem able to get out the words. I asked her to repeat, "red, twenty-three, and Sherbrooke." She did, but in a labored, halting voice. I took her pulse, which bounded at 160 beats per minute. The nurse measured Kim's blood pressure at 126/68 mmHg. Within three minutes, she could speak normally, but began to cry. She continued trembling for another 10 minutes.

After the spell, we measured her blood sugar with the glucometer and it was 86 mg/dl. By the time we got the electrocardiogram hooked up, her heart rate had returned to 75. She was in normal sinus rhythm. We drew blood for a serum prolactin level and sent it to the lab. I kept her in the hospital another day to collect a 24-hour urine for vanillyl-mandelic acid (VMA) and 5-hydroxyindoleacetic acid (5-HIAA) and to obtain a baseline prolactin level the next morning.

Kim's EEG tracings for both spells were normal. I told her she didn't have epilepsy. She promised to follow up with her psychiatrist. I asked her to see me in a month. Prolactin and urine tests were normal.

Questions

109. Does Kim have nonepileptic seizures?

Yes.

Many patients have spells that may be mistaken for epileptic seizures. These may be called pseudoseizures, hysterical seizures, psychogenic seizures, or nonepileptic seizures (NES). Most of these terms imply a psychological underpinning of these spells, which usually is the case. The term *nonepileptic seizure* is preferable, because it includes both organic and psychological events and carries no pejorative connotation.

A small minority of these paroxysmal events represent physiologic problems such as hypoglycemia, syncope, tics, transient global amnesia, transient ischemic attack, or other organic cause. Consequently, each patient must be carefully evaluated to determine the nature of the clinical event.

Monitoring a patient with a video camera and continuous electroencephalographic (EEG) monitoring allows one to study the details of a representative episode. Digital technology for this purpose is now available for inpatient, outpatient, or home monitoring.

Some patients require hospitalization for close observation and to ensure that technical problems do not interfere with the recordings. However, removing patients from their homes to the security of the hospital setting often decreases seizure frequency. This phenomenon is not well understood, but it occurs with both epileptic and nonepileptic seizures. Monitoring patients at home can be more productive, because they are more likely to continue having their typical spells. Outpatient monitoring also is less expensive.

110. Are nonepileptic seizures common?

They are in tertiary epilepsy centers.

One of the distinguishing features of nonepileptic seizures is that antiepileptic drugs (AEDs) fail to control them. Consequently, physicians often refer these patients to epilepsy centers because of "intractable epilepsy." Video-EEG monitoring usually is necessary to make the diagnosis.

Specialists ultimately diagnose approximately 10 percent to 20 percent of patients referred for treatment of uncontrolled seizures with NES. However, nonepileptic seizures may be even more common. In a recent paper presented at the American Academy of Neurology, 55.1 percent of patients referred to an epilepsy monitoring unit had NES. Only 36.5 percent had epilepsy!

It is difficult to know how many people have NES. Approximately 5 percent of patients have both epileptic seizures and nonepileptic seizures. From this number we can calculate a low estimate of the number of patients with NES.

If we assume 1 of 200 people with epilepsy, multiplied by 5 percent of people with both epilepsy and NES, times 250,000,000 citizens of the United States, we arrive at 62,500 people with NES and epilepsy. Many others have NES alone. Nonepileptic seizures should be suspected when patients fail to respond to appropriate therapy.

111. Who is at risk for nonepileptic seizures?

The high-risk group consists of young adult women.

Approximately 75 percent of patients with NES are women. Most of these patients present between the ages of 15 to 35. A history of sexual abuse may be related to this female preponderance.

Nonepileptic seizures also occur in infants, children, and the elderly. Some spells are not psychological in origin, but rather represent misinterpretation of particular behaviors. Here are several examples.

Masturbation in infants can involve rhythmic back arching, rocking, and pelvic thrusting, and has been mistaken for seizures. Other infant behaviors may resemble epileptic seizures. I reviewed a video of an infant receiving antiepileptic medication for uncontrolled seizures. The child had benign head banging (Jactatio capitis).

An 8-year-old with well-controlled convulsions came to our center because his mother noticed a different type of seizure during his sleep. Video-EEG monitoring revealed benign sleep myoclonus, and we reassured her that his seizures were controlled.

One elderly patient came to me for treatment of partial complex seizures. He had peculiar behaviors, such as repeatedly folding a handkerchief and shaving the same part of his face over and over again. Video-EEG monitoring did not reveal any epileptic activity, and we attributed these events to dementia, not epilepsy.

One of my patients who worked in a local shipyard received a blow to the head from a boat deck as it was lowered to fit into its hull. He got up and continued to work, but the next day he had a severe headache and passed out. Over the next two weeks, his very concerned fiancée noticed several episodes in which he seemed to be in a trance and did not respond to her frequent questions. She thought he was having seizures.

His neurologic examination, magnetic resonance imaging scan, EEG, and ambulatory EEG monitoring were all normal. Eventually it became clear that his spells were benign episodes of inattention. They were unrelated to the head injury.

In all of these examples, the "seizures" were in the eye of the beholder.

112. Are there any clinical features in the history that suggest nonepileptic seizures?

Yes, but none are diagnostic.

The wide variety of true epileptic seizures combined with the imprecise history provided by most patients and witnesses makes the diagnosis of NES by history a precarious endeavor. Nonetheless, certain clues raise one's index of suspicion. Enough of these clues in the same patient warrants referral for epilepsy monitoring and psychiatric assessment.

- Seizures do not respond to appropriate AEDs
- Multiple seizure types
- Emotional triggers
- Occur only in presence of others
- Exposure to epileptic seizures
- "La belle indifference"
- Prior psychiatric history
- History of sexual abuse

As discussed in Chapter 2, monotherapy controls seizures in 70 percent of patients with epilepsy. Consequently, when a patient fails to respond to an AED, one must question whether the patient has resistant epilepsy or another disorder or illness.

Many patients with epilepsy exhibit multiple seizure types. A patient may have partial simple seizures with olfactory auras, partial complex seizures with staring and automatisms, and generalized tonic-clonic convulsions. On the other hand, some patients with NES have too many seizure types. Sometimes their hands tremble, sometimes their body shakes, other times they stare, their left eye twitches uncontrollably, once in a while they have tingling down their right side. . . . There is a point at which an excess of symptoms leads away from the diagnosis of epilepsy rather than toward it.

Although patients with epilepsy may relate seizures to periods of increased stress, epileptic seizures rarely occur in the middle of an argument or other confrontation. It is striking how often patients have nonepileptic seizures during morning rounds or when families visit. Events commonly occur just after a physician or family member leaves the patient's room. It seemed strangely fortuitous that Kim had her "big seizure" immediately after I left, particularly because she typically has spells only twice a month and had just had one the day before. Similarly, some patients have seizures only when an audience is present to appreciate them.

Many patients with NES have a "model" for their seizures. I saw one woman whose daughter had cerebral palsy and lived in a residential care center. This woman had witnessed countless seizures and their dramatic effects on observers. Patients may have friends or relatives who serve as models. Kim studied psychology and works in a psychiatric hospital where she has witnessed epileptic convulsions. What began for Kim as simple panic attacks have evolved into more complex phenomena mistaken for epileptic seizures.

Certain patients with NES exhibit an odd demeanor termed "la belle indifference" regarding their spells. Most patients with epilepsy express intense concern about seizures that prevent them from driving, threaten their employment, and cause embarrassment and injuries. Some patients with NES relate stories of multiple ER visits, loss of driving privileges, minor injuries, and relentless seizures despite receiving multiple AEDs with a surprisingly calm and detached manner—as if all of these problems really had no importance. This impressive incongruence between symptom severity and the patient's casual disregard suggests a conversion disorder.

With her new job, marital problems, concerns about her father, and disruptive seizures, Kim appears to have many psychosocial stressors. Yet, when I examined her, she seemed nonchalant and relatively untroubled. This presentation represents either an extraordinary amount of forced composure or, more likely, an example of "la belle indifference."

A prior psychiatric history is common in patients with pseudoseizures. Since she started college, Kim has experienced intermittent symptoms of shortness of breath, dizziness, tachycardia, trembling, shaking, and feelings of unreality—all symptoms of panic disorder. Her parents suddenly separated when she reached puberty, which raises the issue of possible paternal sexual abuse. She also has struggled with an eating disorder that appears to be under control.

Two of my patients had a history of unexplained paralysis of both lower extremities, which required hospitalization. Symptoms spontaneously resolved, probably representing conversion disorders. Inexplicable sensory alterations on the limbs and face are often detected on examination in patients with NES. Chronic pain, depression, sexual abuse, suicide attempts, and substance abuse are common in patients with NES. However, patients with epilepsy also have an increased incidence of psychiatric problems (see Chapter 7).

113. Are there any distinguishing clinical characteristics of nonepileptic seizures?

Yes, but as with the clinical history, none are diagnostic.

Nonepileptic seizures take many shapes and forms, from staring spells to convulsive-like activity. They can be as protean as epileptic seizures. However, NES may possess characteristics atypical for epileptic seizures.

- Gradual onset
- Gradual offset
- Last too long
- Precipitated by suggestion
- No involvement of face
- Thrashing movements
- Pelvic thrusting
- Opisthotonic posturing
- Directed motor activity
- Resist eye opening
- Crying
- Lack of postictal period
- Lack of self-injury

Most epileptic seizures occur fairly abruptly. Even those that are preceded by auras come on within seconds. Nonepileptic seizures often initiate over minutes, so slowly that it is a common conundrum to determine exactly when a seizure begins.

Kim's spell had a very gradual onset. She had time to tell the secretary that she was having a seizure, then went to her supervisor's office to get her doctor's phone number. Most partial complex seizures would not permit this kind of sustained motor and cognitive activity.

Similarly, NES may end gradually, with diminishing symptoms over a number of minutes. Kim's spell in the hospital did not appear to be over until she could speak fluently, finished crying, and stopped trembling.

Epileptic seizures rarely last longer than two minutes, whereas nonepileptic seizures often last much longer. In one study, epileptic seizures always lasted less than 92 seconds, but nonepileptic seizures lasted up to 800 seconds. After Kim regained the ability to speak, she continued to tremble for another 10 minutes. Symptoms of this duration would be atypical for a partial complex seizure.

Nonepileptic seizures often can be precipitated by suggestion. Various "activation" or "induction" procedures can be used, including hyperventilation, sleep deprivation, alcohol swabs applied to the neck, a tuning fork placed on the forehead, IV injection of normal saline ("Actisol"), and an intensive psychiatric interview. The physician combines one or more of these maneuvers with convincing suggestion that a seizure is likely to appear. In order not to "trick" the patient, the physician must enlist the patient's cooperation to try to provoke the typical spell in order to make an accurate diagnosis and begin the proper treatment. In this therapeutic paradigm, the activation procedure becomes a positive part of the doctor-patient relationship.

Some patients report particular triggers for their seizures. One woman claimed that she had spells only while vacuuming, so we procured a vacuum cleaner for her to use in her hospital room. A stationary bicycle or rowing machine can be used for patients who find that exercise precipitates spells. (Patients must be supervised while using these machines. A reclining bicycle is preferable to avoid falls.)

Patients can have convulsive-like episodes that oddly spare the face. There is no blinking or grimacing. This nonphysiologic presentation suggests NES.

Wild thrashing in bed with kicking or flailing suggests either a frontal lobe seizure or NES. The latter are more common. Unfortunately, the EEG often is obscured during these spells because of movement artifact. Diagnosis can be difficult.

Opisthotonus typical of a hysterical convulsion was described in the nineteenth century by the Salpêtrière physicians and illustrated as "arc en cercle." This dramatic posturing still occurs in some patients with NES. (Opisthotonus also may rarely occur as part of the immediate postictal phase of an epileptic tonic-clonic convulsion.)

A confident observation of directed motor activity during a convulsion strongly suggests NES. One of my patients, the newly married wife of a handsome police officer, kicked her solicitous husband through the bed rails as she thrashed about for an hour. Although this kick appeared accidental, it was followed almost immediately by a second, more directed, forceful kick. To further clarify the nature of her "convulsion," the patient abruptly stopped "seizing" to answer the ringing bedside telephone.

Patients with nonepileptic seizures often resist eye opening, whereas patients with epileptic seizures do not. Similarly, NES patients may also avoid a limb dropped in the direction of their face.

Kim cried during her seizure at work, and also after the one I witnessed in the hospital. Ictal lacrimation is exceedingly rare. An emotional release after a seizure almost always indicates NES related to significant psychological issues.

Although patients with absence seizures may resume their conversation immediately after a seizure exactly where they left off, patients with partial complex seizures or generalized tonic-clonic seizures typically have a postictal state characterized by fatigue and confusion. A prolonged convulsion without a postictal state, as in the case of the police officer's wife, raises suspicions of NES.

During an event, patients with NES may bite their tongues or lips, become incontinent, or injure themselves. Injury occurs more commonly in epileptic seizures, but does not eliminate the possibility of nonepileptic seizures.

In order to make an accurate diagnosis, it is critical to witness the patient's typical spell. If necessary for confirmation, the video can be shown to a family member or friend. If patients have more than one type of spell, both or all must be recorded. Patients may have two types of nonepileptic seizures, or may have nonepileptic seizures and epileptic seizures.

114. Can the EEG reliably differentiate epileptic from nonepileptic seizures?

Most of the time.

Twenty percent to 30 percent of patients with epilepsy have a normal EEG between seizures. Conversely, a number of patients with NES, like Kim, have an abnormal EEG. An abnormal EEG may result from prior birth injury, static encephalopathy, head injury, encephalitis, or many other causes. Kim's childhood head injury may have produced nonspecific slowing reported as "abnormal" by the neurologist (see Resource Z).

One should not be misled by interictal EEG recordings. Recording the EEG during a spell provides the most useful information.

The ictal EEG does not always confirm the diagnosis. Muscle artifact resulting from patient movement may obscure epileptic activity in patients with major motor seizures and can frustrate diagnostic efforts. Some patients remove electrodes during the night and sabotage the recording. Epileptic activity from partial simple seizures may not be detected by scalp electrodes. More sensitive monitoring with depth or grid electrodes is too invasive for routine evaluation of suspected NES.

My partner's father came to me with intermittent tingling of his right index finger, which occurred several times a week. Magnetic resonance imaging identified a small infarct in the left middle cerebral artery territory. Electroencephalographic monitoring during these events, which could have been partial simple seizures or transient ischemic attacks, failed to reveal epileptic activity. Aspirin therapy did not prevent the symptoms. Clinically, the spells appeared to be partial simple seizures resulting from the prior infarct. The spells disappeared on a low dose of phenytoin, which suggests that they were epileptic seizures, despite the normal EEG.

Video-EEG provides an accurate diagnosis for most patients. The presence of epileptic activity during a spell is conclusive. The absence of epileptic activity is more problematic and must be interpreted in the clinical context.

115. Can a prolactin level help confirm the diagnosis of epilepsy?

Yes.

The anterior pituitary gland produces prolactin hormone. Serum prolactin levels increase after approximately 90 percent of generalized tonic-clonic seizures and 70 percent of partial complex seizures.

In cases in which the EEG is unclear, a prolactin level drawn within 20 minutes of a seizure and compared with a baseline level drawn 24 hours later can be useful. The level should increase to at least double the baseline before it is considered significant.

Prolactin levels are less valuable for other seizure types. Partial simple seizures and partial complex frontal lobe seizures often do not produce prolactin elevations. Absence, akinetic, and myoclonic seizures do not raise prolactin. Prolactin levels may not be elevated in status epilepticus.

Because prolactin levels vary throughout the day, a baseline level is required. Confounding factors that elevate prolactin levels include haloperidol, phenothiazines, pregnancy, lactation, and prolactinomas.

116. Are there any other etiologies for nonepileptic seizures besides psychological problems?

Yes.

The vast majority of nonepileptic seizures are due to psychological problems. However, neurologic and nonneurologic etiologies may also be responsible for unexplained spells and warrant a thorough medical evaluation.

Alcoholic blackouts, benign myoclonus, hyperekplexia, hypoglycemia, periodic movements of sleep, paroxysmal kinesigenic dyskinesia, syncope, transient global amnesia, and transient ischemic attacks are some of the physiologic causes of NES (see question 111).

One of my female patients with diabetes would suddenly slump over without warning. Her spells had a "swooning" quality to them, but they were not believed to be syncope because they also occurred while she was supine. Close observation of these spells revealed episodes of hypotension related to severe diabetic autonomic neuropathy.

A young man had repeated episodes of flushing and syncope. Extensive cardiac and metabolic workups were negative. Finally, bone marrow examination revealed evidence of systemic mastocytosis. His spells resulted from massive histamine release.

Two of my patients had episodes in which they would appear drowsy and lose consciousness, but they denied fatigue. Video-EEG monitoring revealed that they simply fell asleep. The patients did not recognize that they were tired.

Because of Kim's paroxysmal tachycardia, I ordered 24-hour urine studies for vanillylmandelic acid (VMA) and 5-hydroxyindoleacetic acid (5-HIAA) to make sure she didn't have a pheochromocytoma or carcinoid tumor. She didn't. Thyroid studies were also normal.

117. Should patients with suspected nonepileptic seizures have a psychological evaluation?

Yes.

A neuropsychologist and psychiatrist are critical components of the epilepsy team. Patients with epilepsy often have psychological problems, as do most patients with NES. An interview by a neuropsychologist or psychiatrist often elicits revealing psychosocial history. In some patients with NES, neuropsychological testing such as the Minnesota Multiphasic Personality Inventory reveals a profile with hypochondriasis and hysteria elevations and a low depression score.

Psychological evaluation can provide a basis for subsequent psychotherapy. Identification of symptoms such as anxiety or depression may lead to specific medication treatment.

118. Is there any role for antiepileptic medications in the treatment of nonepileptic seizures?

No.

As discussed elsewhere (see Chapter 6), AEDs are not benign agents. The one case of Dilantin hypersensitivity syndrome I have seen occurred in a patient referred with intractable epilepsy who actually had NES. In addition, AEDs have been observed to worsen, rather than improve NES.

I do not favor using AEDs as a therapeutic trial for unexplained seizures. If the seizures stop, there is a strong possibility of a placebo response. This route has the unfortunate consequences of labeling the patient with the diagnosis of epilepsy and needlessly exposing the patient to AED side effects. In addition, it makes it very difficult to decide when to stop using the AED (see Chapter 3).

When patients have both epilepsy and nonepileptic seizures, AEDs treat the epilepsy.

One must make a definitive diagnosis as soon as possible in order to direct therapy at the underlying cause of the patient's spells and spare the patient the expense and risk of inappropriate therapies. Concerns of drug toxicity are particularly acute in this group of patients because the majority are women of childbearing age.

119. Are nonepileptic seizures likely to get better?

It depends on the etiology.

For some patients with NES, merely explaining the diagnosis and providing reassurance that the troubling spells do not represent epilepsy results in a cure.

Other patients reluctantly accept the diagnosis of NES. However, once epilepsy has been eliminated as the cause of their spells, the patients can direct their attention to stressful circumstances in their lives. These patients describe overwhelming psychosocial stressors, including sexual abuse, financial ruin, lost homes, litigation, and severe marital and other personal problems. Nonepileptic seizures often develop in people with limited insight and coping abilities, qualities that confound treatment. The physician can sympathetically view these somatic symptoms as a "cry for help" and assist the patient in obtaining neuropsychological and psychiatric intervention.

Very few patients with NES deliberately stage their spells (malinger). More commonly, the spells represent a conversion disorder, where the patient is not conscious of the underlying psychological etiology. Consequently, patients often become offended or angry when accused of "faking" their seizures.

Whereas many people object to being labeled with a psychiatric diagnosis, few deny that "stress" plays an important role in their lives. Most people concede that stress can produce headaches. From that analogy, it is not much of a stretch to suggest that stress can underlie other neurologic symptoms, such as abnormal body movements or staring spells. Patients often accept this line of reasoning.

If the patient does not have epilepsy, AEDs should be slowly withdrawn and the patient should be counseled to refrain from rushing to the ER when a spell occurs. Frequently, with the full history unavailable, the ER physician will restart AEDs and unknowingly perpetuate the patient's lingering belief that the spells represent epilepsy. (One of my patients had her carbamazepine restarted three times as a result of repeated visits to the ER.)

In addition to treatment by a neuropsychologist and psychiatrist, I have found that there are beneficial effects to seeing patients with NES in a monthly therapy group. The sessions validate the patients' illness, allow them to meet others who have the same problem, and provide a scheduled opportunity for them to address their concerns to the doctor. Some of these patients have spent years as "neurology patients" and reject the idea of seeing a psychiatrist. These sessions provide an opportunity to continue to educate patients about NES and direct their care.

Patients who have a history of NES longer than one year, personality disorder, or Munchausen syndrome tend to have a poor prognosis.

Recommendations for treatment:

- Accurate diagnosis
- Acknowledge there is a problem (even if it is not "neurologic")
- Present the diagnosis therapeutically—"good news, you don't have epilepsy, but these spells represent a significant stress in your life"
- Taper and withdraw AEDs
- Educate patient and family to avoid going to ER
- Refer for psychotherapy to learn coping skills, insight
- Refer for psychiatric evaluation for possible treatment of depression, anxiety, or other psychiatric disorder
- Refer to a social worker—many of these patients have significant social concerns regarding finances, transportation, employment, housing, and so forth
- Reassurance, care for the patient
- Team approach—neurologist, neuropsychologist, psychiatrist, and social worker

12

Alternative Therapy

John is an 81-year-old man whose seizures began at the age of 64. No convincing etiology for his epilepsy had ever been identified. His seizures were difficult to control. I met him after he fell on an icy sidewalk and developed a traumatic quadriparesis from central cord syndrome. Luckily, his symptoms improved dramatically after a few days of immobilization. His only residua were mild numbness of his left hand, a slightly stiff gait, and bilateral brisk reflexes.

Seizures occurred every few weeks. He became disoriented, chewed, rocked in his chair, and occasionally developed a tonic-clonic seizure. John functioned independently despite a number of other medical problems, including chronic anemia, diverticulosis, hypertension, leukopenia, severe osteoarthritis, prostate cancer, and mild memory loss. He took hydrochlorothiazide, ibuprofen, leuprolide, potassium, and multivitamins.

Before I met him, he had tried carbamazepine, divalproex sodium, phenytoin, and phenobarbital. I added topiramate to his carbamazepine. His wife expressed concern that the trauma of another convulsion could result in further spinal cord injury. She sighed when I told her it would take a month or two to increase the topiramate to its optimal dosage.

John's computed axial tomography (CAT) scan was normal. His magnetic resonance imaging (MRI) scan revealed mild generalized cerebral atrophy and diffuse ischemic white matter disease. His electroencephalogram showed bilateral independent temporal spikes. In addition to the antiepileptic drugs (AEDs), his wife gave him large doses of shark cartilage. At our last visit, she insisted that I endorse this alternative treatment and encourage John to take the white powder with his prescription medication.

117

Questions

120. Has shark cartilage been proven helpful for epilepsy?

No.

When one reviews the multitude of natural compounds that have been tried in the treatment of epilepsy, it is not surprising that shark cartilage should be included. Sharks have roamed the seas for millions of years, have no natural enemies, eat everything from license plates to humans, appear disease resistant, and mysteriously have no bones. That's quite a résumé to attract public attention and wonder.

Shark cartilage has become popular for the treatment of cancer and osteoporosis. Sold as a food supplement, it has not been approved by the U.S. Food and Drug Administration (FDA) for the treatment of anything. (At present, one cannot conclude that shark cartilage is useless, only that it has not been proven useful.)

The episodic nature of epilepsy complicates its treatment. Patients may appear to be cured, only to have another seizure weeks or months later. Remedies derived from seal genitals, hippopotamus testicles, tortoise blood, crocodile feces, mistletoe, and gladiator liver have not withstood the test of time.

Treatment is also confounded by those patients who have syndromes that resemble epilepsy, ranging from syncope to pseudoseizures. To adequately evaluate novel therapies, well-designed, double-blind, placebo controlled trials must be performed in large numbers of patients who carry a secure diagnosis. This type of methodical, dispassionate clinical trial is a relatively new phenomenon in the history of epilepsy treatment.

121. Does shark cartilage interfere with the metabolism of topiramate?

I don't know.

The answer to this question is important, and I don't know what it is. Looking up "shark cartilage" under drug interactions in the *Physician's Desk Reference* or contacting the medical affairs office at Ortho-McNeil is unlikely to provide the answer.

One of my frustrations with novel therapies is that I cannot reassure patients that the new treatment won't interfere with my prescribed medication. There already are significant dosing considerations for John's AEDs. Because of his age and corresponding decreased renal clearance, he requires a slightly lower topiramate dose. On the other hand, his topiramate dose needs to be higher because he takes carbamazepine, a potent enzyme inducer. If I taper the carbamazepine, I will have to reduce the topiramate dose to keep its level constant. These considerations are detailed in the package insert.

Where does shark cartilage fit into these delicate pharmacokinetic considerations? The answers are not available.

122. What about calcium and magnesium supplements?

No evidence of benefit.

Patients often confuse medical literature regarding mineral deficiencies with the value of supplements. Although it is well documented that hypocalcemia and hypomagnesemia can result in seizures, there is no evidence that calcium and magnesium supplements prevent seizures when no deficiency exists.

123. What about vitamin supplements?

No evidence of benefit.

Vitamin supplementation is essential in the exceedingly rare condition of pyridoxine (vitamin B6) deficiency. This condition usually is seen in infants. Otherwise, there is no evidence that any vitamin supplements control seizures.

124. Is there a role for hormone therapy in the treatment of adults with epilepsy?

Only in very experienced hands.

Estrogen lowers the seizure threshold, whereas progesterone decreases epileptiform discharges (see Chapter 5). Some women have catamenial epilepsy, a condition in which seizure frequency is linked to the menstrual cycle. Seizures occur less often when progesterone levels are highest, during the luteal phase. Because of these observations, a variety of hormonal manipulations have been attempted in efforts at seizure control.

Natural progesterone has helped some women with catamenial epilepsy. Multiple side effects of progesterone, including breast tenderness, weight gain, and irregular vaginal bleeding, limit this treatment. Parenteral synthetic progestin in doses high enough to produce amenorrhea can improve seizure control. Clomiphene can improve seizure frequency in women with a documented inadequate luteal phase. A small number of women improved on triptorelin, a synthetic gonadotropin-releasing hormone analogue. (John is taking leuprolide, a gonadotropin-releasing hormone agonist, for his prostate cancer. It does not appear to help his seizures.)

Metabolic factors related to hormonal cycles may play a role in seizure frequency as well. Some women experience an increase in seizures just before menstruation. Sex hormones and AEDs compete for the same hepatic microsomal enzymes. The premenstrual decline in gonadal steroid secretion may allow increased hepatic metabolism of AEDs, resulting in lower AED levels and increased seizures.

Testosterone therapy has not been reported to control seizures in men. In one case report, clomiphene improved seizure control and sexual performance in a man with hypogonadotropic hypogonadism.

Case reports and small studies suggest that hormone supplementation can improve seizure control in selected patients. Significant side effects may occur, including hot flashes, headaches, and pregnancy. Patients must carefully track their menstrual cycle and seizure occurrence on a calendar. Hormonal therapy is not approved for the treatment of adult epilepsy and is best performed under the supervision of a neuroendocrinologist when conventional treatments fail.

Note: Adrenocorticotropic hormone (ACTH) has been used since the 1950s for the treatment of West syndrome, a triad of infantile spasms, mental retardation, and the distinctive EEG pattern of hypsarrhythmia. Approximately 25 percent of these infants have tuberous sclerosis. Although the best therapy for West syndrome remains under investigation, many pediatric neurologists recommend ACTH for this condition. ACTH is not approved for adults with epilepsy.

125. Can behavioral therapy be useful?

Yes.

On the most basic level, appropriate behavioral therapy involves modifying behavior to achieve 100 percent compliance with medication and office visits, lifestyle adjustment to ensure adequate sleep and nutrition, and avoidance of epileptogenic precipitants such as heroin and cocaine.

More specifically, patients with reflex epilepsy can identify triggers that provoke seizures such as photic stimulation or reading. Changing behavior to avoid these stimuli can reduce seizure frequency. Wearing special polarizing glasses may suppress a photoparoxysmal response. I had one patient with reading epilepsy who felt his face begin to twitch after he read for about 15 minutes. This was the partial motor component of his seizure. If he stopped reading at that moment, he could prevent the twitching from evolving into a generalized tonic-clonic seizure. He learned to do this and rarely had a convulsion.

Some patients abort seizures when they have an aura by stimulating a specific area of the body. For example, if a patient has a sensory aura in an arm, squeezing the arm with the other hand may prevent the seizure from progressing. Similarly, a patient with an olfactory aura may counteract it with a strong olfactory stimulus. Some patients insist that "concentrating" aborts seizures. Although these methods may be helpful, they usually are not reliable.

Many patients report "stress" as an inciting factor for seizures. Stress management techniques and exercise may help patients reduce seizure frequency.

126. Is it common for patients to resort to alternative medicine?

Yes.

"Alternative medicine" may be viewed as treatments that have not entered mainstream Western medicine. They have not been scientifically proven. (If they were proven useful, they would immediately be accepted by physicians and would no longer fall into the category of "alternative medicine"!)

In one survey, more than 28 percent of family practice patients used alternative medicine. These patients tended to be female and well-educated. Acupuncture, herbal therapy, massage therapy, and chiropractic treatment were the most common methods. Pain and stress were the main indications. Eighty-two percent reported some improvement, but less than 50 percent were completely satisfied. Most patients did not tell their doctors about using these additional treatments.

Extraordinary sums are spent each year on unproven alternative therapies. In 1996, Americans spent 3.24 billion dollars for herbal medications alone. Because of widespread interest and use of alternative therapies, the Office of Alternative Medicine, a division of the National Institutes of Health, is systematically evaluating some of these treatments. In 1998 the Office of Alternative Medicine had a budget of $20 million.

Many alternative medicine practitioners are physicians, particularly generalists, family physicians, and psychiatrists. More than 50 percent of physicians refer patients for alternative therapy.

John's wife is unsatisfied with his treatment, and rightfully so. Despite trials of four AEDs, and now with the addition of a fifth, he still has seizures. A severe convulsion could result in another devastating episode of paralysis. Furthermore, no clear etiology for his seizure disorder has emerged despite multiple EEGs, an expensive MRI scan, and a CAT scan. John also had a two-day evaluation by a neuropsychologist, who confirmed the symptoms of memory loss but had little to offer to help treat them.

John's wife is frustrated, and so am I. Unfortunately, there is no convincing evidence that shark cartilage will improve John's health, and I don't have enough information on its safety to endorse it. Hippocrates recommended that epilepsy be treated with "diet and drugs," and "not by magic." At the moment, shark cartilage falls into the latter category.

127. Does the medical literature validate any alternative treatments for epilepsy?

No.

Although there are occasional favorable reports, there is no body of evidence to demonstrate effectiveness of epilepsy treatment for the following alternative therapies: acupuncture, amulets, bracelets, enzyme therapy, foot reflexology, herbal treatments, homeopathy, hypnotherapy, meditation, magnetism, metamorphosis therapy, orthomolecular medicine, spiritual and faith healing, stones, or yoga. With the high interest level in alternative therapies, perhaps formal studies will yield unequivocal results.

Other than AEDs, several other therapeutic approaches control seizures in certain patients. Epilepsy surgery, the vagal nerve stimulator, and the ketogenic diet are discussed in Chapter 2.

128. Is there any danger in using alternative medicine?

Yes.

Most patients use alternative medicine treatments in conjunction with traditional therapies, making them "complementary" therapies rather than "alternative" ones. This distinction is important, because much of the harm of alternative therapies comes from their exclusive use. Patients put themselves at risk when they abandon conventional therapies that, although suboptimal, may be helpful. For example, some patients who put their faith in "spiritual healing" and stopped taking their AEDs ended up in the hospital with status epilepticus.

Another significant risk is delay to medical treatment. I saw one teenaged boy about a year after his seizures began, whose mother had treated him with herbs grown in her own garden. She was convinced that this natural treatment would be far superior to anything modern medicine had to offer. After his sixth emergency room (ER) visit for convulsions, she finally took the ER doctor's advice and brought her son for a neurologic evaluation.

The boy had myoclonic jerks when he was fatigued, and occasional tonic-clonic seizures. He was a bright, talented young man, who had a normal neurologic examination. His EEG revealed generalized spike and wave. His mother also had seizures. She took phenytoin, but didn't like its side effects. His was a straightforward case of myoclonic epilepsy of Janz, and I had every reason to believe that a low dose of valproate would control his seizures.

His mother may have had the same diagnosis and would have benefited from a change in medication, but she never consented to an evaluation. The boy could have been spared the medical and psychological impact of a year of uncontrolled seizures and his mother could have avoided thousands of dollars of ER bills if she had taken him to a neurologist sooner.

Yet another concern is the potential toxicity of ingested compounds. The FDA does not regulate food supplements in the same manner as prescription medications. The potency and purity of preparations vary widely. Patients may be allergic to certain ingredients. Megadoses of fat-soluble vitamins can be toxic.

In the last 20 years more than 100 deaths can be attributed to herbal "remedies." Complications requiring renal dialysis, renal transplantation, and liver transplantation have occurred.

In addition, herbal preparations, such as "herbal ecstasy" or Ma Huang, which contains ephedrine, have been reported to precipitate seizures. Hemolysis can result from "green water" used by the Celestial Church.

Patients spend billions of dollars for acupuncture, vitamins, herbs, shark cartilage, and other unproven treatments. Unfortunately, these financial investments are based on hope, unproven theories, appealing anecdotes, and desperation, *not* on evidence-based medicine. As research continues into both conventional and unconventional treatments, we will have more to offer our patients and their money will be better spent. In the meantime, *Primum Non Nocere.*

Resources

**International Classification of Epilepsies and
Epileptic Syndromes
(condensed)**

I. Localization-related (focal, local, partial) epilepsies and syndromes
   1.1 Idiopathic (age-related onset)
   - Benign childhood epilepsy with centrotemporal spikes
   - Childhood epilepsy with occipital paroxysms
   - Primary reading epilepsy
   1.2 Symptomatic
   - Chronic progressive epilepsia partialis continua of childhood (Kojewnikow's syndrome)
   - Syndromes characterized by seizures with specific modes of precipitation
   - Temporal lobe epilepsies
   - Frontal lobe epilepsies
   - Parietal lobe epilepsies
   - Occipital lobe epilepsies
   1.3 Cryptogenic

II. Generalized epilepsies and syndromes
   2.1 Idiopathic (age-related onset)
   - Benign neonatal familial convulsions
   - Benign neonatal convulsions
   - Benign myoclonic epilepsy in infancy

- Childhood absence epilepsy (pyknolepsy)
- Juvenile absence epilepsy
- Juvenile myoclonic epilepsy
- Epilepsy with grand mal seizures on awakening
- Other
- Epilepsies with seizures precipitated by specific modes of activation

2.2 Cryptogenic or symptomatic
- West syndrome
- Lennox-Gastaut syndrome
- Epilepsy with myoclonic-astatic seizures
- Epilepsy with myoclonic absences

2.3 Symptomatic
- Early myoclonic encephalopathy
- Early infantile epileptic encephalopathy with suppression burst
- Other
- Epileptic seizures complicating other disease states

III. Epilepsies and syndromes undetermined whether focal or generalized
- Neonatal seizures
- Severe myoclonic epilepsy in infancy
- Epilepsy with continuous spike-waves during slow wave sleep
- Acquired epileptic aphasia (Landau-Kleffner syndrome)
- Other

IV. Special syndromes
- Febrile convulsions
- Isolated seizures or isolated status epilepticus
- Seizures due to metabolic or toxic provocation such as alcohol, drugs, or eclampsia

Resource B

International Classification of Epileptic Seizures (condensed)

I. Partial (Focal, Local) Seizures
    A. Simple partial seizures
    B. Complex partial seizures
       1. With impairment of consciousness at onset
       2. Simple partial onset followed by impairment of consciousness
    C. Partial seizures evolving to generalized tonic-clonic convulsions (GTC)
       1. Simple evolving to GTC
       2. Complex evolving to GTC

II. Generalized Seizures (Convulsive or Nonconvulsive)
    A. 1. Absence
       2. Atypical absence
    B. Myoclonic
    C. Clonic
    D. Tonic
    E. Tonic-clonic
    F. Atonic

III. Unclassified

Resource C
Seizure History Checklist

- Difficult birth?
- Premature?
- Multiple birth?
- Low birth weight?
- Prolonged hospital stay?
- Delayed speech?
- Delayed walking?
- Completed high school?
- Completed college?
- Special classes?
- Family member with epilepsy?
- Febrile seizures?
- Encephalitis?
- Meningitis?
- Head injury with loss of consciousness?
- Warning before seizure?
- Staring spell?
- Convulsion?
- Incontinence?
- Tongue biting?
- Postictal fatigue?
- Postictal headache?
- Postictal confusion?
- Seizure frequency?
- Seizures at time of menses?
- Seizures only at night?
- Seizures only in morning?
- Seizure triggers?

Resource D

Drug Information
Brand Names, Generic Names, and Abbreviations

Celontin	methsuximide	MSM
Cerebyx	fosphenytoin	PHT
Dilantin	phenytoin	PHT
Depakene	valproic acid	VPA
Depakote	divalproex sodium	DVS
Diamox	acetazolamide	AZM
Felbatol	felbamate	FBM
Gabitril	tiagabine	TG
Keppra	levetiracetam	LEV
Klonopin	clonazepam	CZP
Lamictal	lamotrigine	LTG
Mebaral	mephobarbital	MPB
Mysoline	primidone	PRM
Neurontin	gabapentin	GBP
Phenobarbital	phenobarbital	PB
Tegretol	carbamazepine	CBZ
Topamax	topiramate	TPM
Tranxene	clorazepate	CLZ
Trileptal	oxcarbazepine	OXC
Zarontin	ethosuximide	ESM

Resource E

Antiepileptic Drugs in Development

Brand Name	Generic
pending	flunarazine
pending	ganaxolone
pending	harkoseride
pending	loreclezole
pending	losigamone
pending	piracetam
pending	pregabalin
pending	remacemide
pending	rufinamide
pending	stiripentol
Sabril	vigabatrin
Zonegran*	zonisamide

*Zonegran was issued an approvable letter by the FDA on March 19, 1998.

Comment:

In my neurology practice, I cared for Mary, a 27-year-old woman who had partial complex seizures several times a week. Mild memory impairment caused her to struggle to remember the varying doses and intervals of her ever-changing medication regimen. Her husband helped her and patiently repeated my instructions when she didn't understand them.

In our last session, she asked me very sincerely whether there was any possibility that she would ever be free of her seizures. She had been hoping to control her seizures before becoming pregnant, but she hadn't succeeded. She was afraid to conceive while taking multiple antiepileptic drugs and was totally frustrated by her continued seizures. Not knowing what to do, Mary called her father in Florida. He told her that she had taken fits since she was a little girl, that he and her mother had been to every specialist and tried every medication, and that she would always have seizures. There was no point believing anything else. Mary wanted to know if I thought her case was hopeless, too.

All of us who care for intractable epilepsy patients know that miracles are few and far between. Yet each of us have seen "hopeless" patients become seizure-free, whether through improved compliance, a new medication, or epilepsy surgery.

The investigational drugs listed above represent hope for patients with epilepsy. Each new antiepileptic medication that comes to market represents an enormous effort on the part of willing patients, dedicated clinicians, and competitive pharmaceutical companies. I reminded Mary that she was doing better than ever on the last medication we tried, and many more options were to come. We also discussed a unique nonpharmaceutical treatment, the vagal stimulator.

It is likely that not all of the drugs listed will be approved by the Food and Drug Administration. Some will fail to demonstrate significant efficacy, whereas others will manifest side effects that outweigh their benefit. But some of them will satisfy the rigors of clinical testing, and maybe one will help my patient control her seizures.

Resource F

Conventional Antiepileptic Drugs

Brand Name	Generic Name	Typical Adult Daily Dose	Half-life	Therapeutic Level
Depakote	divalproex sodium	750–3000 mg	6–15 hours	50–150µg/ml
Dilantin	phenytoin	100–400	12–36	10–20
Tegretol	carbamazepine	300–2000	14–27	4–12
Mysoline	primidone	500–1500	6–18	5–12
Phenobarbital	phenobarbital	60–200	40–136	10–40

Resource G
The New Antiepileptic Drugs

Brand Name	Generic Name	Typical Adult Daily Dose	Half-life	Therapeutic Level
Felbatol	felbamate	2400–3600 mg	13–23 hours	32–137 µg/ml
Gabitril	tiagabine	32–56	3–9	5–70 ng/ml (?)
Keppra	levetiracetam	1000–3000 mg	7–10	2.9–60.1 µg/ml
Lamictal monotherapy	lamotrigine	500	25	2–20 µg/ml (?)
Lamictal with enzyme inducers	lamotrigine	300–700	12.6	2–20 µg/ml (?)
Lamictal with valproate	lamotrigine	100–200	58.8	2–20 µg/ml (?)
Lamictal with valproate and enzyme inducers	lamotrigine	100–200	27.2	2–20 µg/ml (?)
Neurontin	gabapentin	900–3600	5–7	4–16 µg/ml (?)
Topamax	topiramate	200–600	12–30	2–25 µg/ml (?)
Trileptal	oxcarbazepine	600–2400	9	4–12 µg/ml (?)

Resource H

Mechanisms of Action of Antiepileptic Drugs*

Brand Name	Generic Name	Reduce Sodium Current	GABA Enhancer	Carbonic Anyhdrase Inhibition	GABA Reuptake Inhibitor	Blocks Calcium Current	Modulates Glutamate Function
Cerebyx	fosphenytoin	X					
Depakene	valproic acid	X	X				
Depakote	divalproex sodium	X	X				
Diamox	acetazolamide			X			
Dilantin	phenytoin	X					
Felbatol	felbamate	X	X			X	X
Gabitril	tiagabine				X		
Keppra†	levetiracetam						
Klonopin	clonazepam		X				
Lamictal	lamotrigine	X					X
Mebaral	mephobarbital	X	X				
Mysoline	primidone	X					
Neurontin	gabapentin		X				
Phenobarbital	phenobarbital	X	X				
Tegretol	carbamazepine	X					
Topamax	topiramate	X	X	X		X	X
Tranzene	clorazepate		X				
Trileptal	oxcarbazepine	X					
Valium	diazepam		X				
Zarontin	ethosuximide					X	

* This table represents a simplified overview of AED mechanisms of action.

† The mechanism(s) of action of Keppra remains unknown.

Resource I

New Preparations of Antiepileptic Drugs

Carbatrol (carbamazepine): Carbatrol is a new formulation of carbamazepine consisting of immediate-release, extended-release, and enteric-release beads. Taken twice a day, Carbatrol provides serum levels comparable to carbamazepine four times a day. This sustained-release preparation reduces toxic serum peaks and ineffective troughs.

Carbatrol may be taken during or between meals. Patients swallow the capsules whole or sprinkle them on food. (Capsules cannot be crushed or chewed.)

The twice-daily dosing facilitates compliance. Side effects and absolute dose are the same as for carbamazepine.

Depacon (valproic acid): Intravenous (IV) Depacon can replace divalproex sodium (Depakote) when patients cannot take medication orally, such as perioperatively or because of nausea and vomiting. The milligram dose remains the same, as Depacon is bioequivalent with divalproex sodium. Depacon should be infused over 60 minutes, but no faster than 20 mg/min. Dizziness (5.2 percent), headache (4.3 percent), nausea (3.2 percent), and injection site pain (2.6 percent) are the most common side effects.

Valproate can cause thrombocytopenia, inhibition of platelet aggregation, and abnormal coagulation tests. Consequently, when Depacon is used perioperatively, one should check platelet count and coagulation parameters. Thrombocytopenia occurs more commonly at serum valproate levels greater than 110 µg/ml (females) and 135 µg/ml (males).

Depacon currently is not indicated for prophylaxis of posttraumatic seizures or status epilepticus. Adverse events of Depacon include those of oral valproate.

Retrospective analysis of hepatic fatalities related to valproate point to children younger than two years old, on multiple antiepileptic drugs (AEDs), with severe seizure disorders, congenital metabolic disorders, mental retardation, and organic brain disease. Valproate should be used cautiously in this group (see Chapter 4, question 32).

Diastat (diazepam): Diastat is a nonsterile diazepam rectal gel indicated for children and adults with intractable epilepsy on stable regimens of AEDs who require treatment for repetitive and predictable seizure clusters. Diastat's main advantage is out-of-hospital administration. If a cluster of seizures can be stopped with rectal diazepam, one can avoid a disruptive and expensive emergency room (ER) visit.

A package insert with instructions and flow chart to record the number of seizures and time of Diastat dose comes with the product. Caregivers need to be trained to recognize seizure clusters and properly administer the drug. After Diastat administration, the patient's respiratory rate and color should be monitored for four hours. Somnolence occurs in almost 25 percent of treated patients. If seizures continue, patients still have the option of going to the ER.

Because of the risk of benzodiazepine drug dependence, Diastat should not be used more than five times per month or every five days. Depending on their age, patients should receive between 0.2 and 0.5 mg/kg/dose.

Tegretol XR (carbamazepine): Tegretol XR is an extended-release tablet that uses the OROS osmotic pump delivery system. An osmotic membrane allows water from the stomach to enter the tablet and dissolve the carbamazepine. The carbamazepine slowly leaks out through a single hole. Because of this special construction, tablets must not be broken, chewed, or crushed.

The tablet coating is not absorbed, and patients may find these film-like capsules in their stools. (Worried patients may bring these specimens to the office for examination unless alerted to expect them.) Patients with short-gut syndrome are difficult to treat with Tegretol XR because the tablet will not have time to release all of its carbamazepine.

Like Carbatrol, patients can be converted from Tegretol or carbamazepine to Tegretol XR on a milligram to milligram basis. Tegretol XR is bioequivalent with Tegretol and its active metabolite, carbamazepine-10,11-epoxide. Side effects are those of carbamazepine.

Cerebyx (fosphenytoin): Fosphenytoin can be administered at a more physiologic pH than phenytoin (8.8 versus 12) and is at least a thousand times more water soluble. (Phenytoin requires 40 percent propylene glycol and 10 percent ethanol to dissolve.) Consequently, fosphenytoin can be given both intravenously (IV) and intramuscularly (IM). Plasma and tissue phosphatases quickly hydrolyze fosphenytoin to phenytoin. The prodrug has a conversion half-life of 8 to 15 minutes.

Fosphenytoin is labeled in phenytoin equivalents (PE) to simplify dosing. The product comes as 50 mg PE/ml concentration in 2 milliliter or 10 milliliter vials.

As with phenytoin, patients require continuous monitoring of blood pressure, respiration, and electrocardiogram during IV infusion. Fosphenytoin can be administered IV at up to 150 mg PE/minute, three times faster than the maximal recommended rate of phenytoin. One can give a complete loading dose for a 70 kg man at 15 mg/kg in seven minutes. Monitoring should be continued for 10 to 20 minutes after the infusion while phosphatases metabolize fosphenytoin to phenytoin. It is best to check phenytoin levels when conversion is complete—two hours after IV infusion and four hours after IM injection.

Transient burning, itching, or tingling commonly accompany IV infusion, but patients tolerate fosphenytoin better than phenytoin. Because phosphate is one of the byproducts of fosphenytoin metabolism, fosphenytoin must be used cautiously in patients with renal failure.

Resource J

Intravenous Antiepileptic Drug Dosing Formulas with Examples

These formulas will help you calculate the correct additional dose of medication for a patient who is known to have a subtherapeutic level of phenytoin or valproate. The goal is to immediately bring the patient's serum level into the therapeutic range with a supplementary intravenous loading dose. In order to use the formula, you must know the patient's weight, current drug level, and volume of distribution of the drug.

Example A

Nancy is an obese 21-year-old woman who had her first seizure one month ago. At that time, she was loaded with phenytoin in the emergency room (ER) and prescribed a daily dose of 100 mg tid. Despite faithfully taking her medication, she arrives by ambulance in the ER at 3:00 in the afternoon, having had a witnessed generalized tonic-clonic seizure at work.

Nancy is disheveled and disoriented in the ER. The left side of her tongue is lacerated where she has bitten it, and her pants are soiled. Over the next hour, the confusion clears and her neurologic examination returns to normal. A stat phenytoin level is 8 µg/ml.

Clearly, Nancy needs to be taking an increased dose of phenytoin. In the meantime, in order to prevent another seizure, it would be prudent to raise her level to the 15–20 µg/ml range. Either traditional phenytoin or the newer fosphenytoin (Cerebyx) can be used (the latter administered in phenytoin equivalents).

The formula is:

$$\text{Dose} = \text{Weight} \times \text{Vd} \times (\text{desired level} - \text{actual level})$$

To use the formula, you need to know that:
1. Vd is the volume of distribution. For phenytoin, the value is 0.7 L/kg

2. Weight is expressed in kilograms

Nancy weighs 160 pounds, or 72.7 kilograms. Her measured level of phenytoin is only 8 µg/ml. It would be better if it were 18 µg/ml. Now we can use the formula:

Dose = 72.7 kg × 0.7 L/kg (18 µg/ml–8 µg/ml)
Dose = 50.89 L × (10 µg/ml)
Dose = 508.9 mg.

According to the formula, if Nancy receives a loading dose of 508.9 mg, her measured level after equilibration will be 18 µg/ml. She receives 500 mg with IV phenytoin over about 10 minutes at 50 mg/minute.

To prevent another breakthrough seizure, her phenytoin dose is increased to 400 mg/day in two divided doses. She is sent home from the ER with instructions to have a serum phenytoin level checked in one week and to follow up with her neurologist.

Note: The dosing formula does not estimate the chronic daily dose, only the one-time dose to augment the serum level.

Example B

Danny is a 30-year-old man with Crohn's disease and well-controlled myoclonic epilepsy of Janz. He typically takes 500 mg bid of divalproex sodium; his levels usually stay at around 70 µg/ml. His last seizure was three years ago. However, he has been hospitalized for an exacerbation of his Crohn's disease and has been NPO for the last 48 hours. He is very concerned about his Depakote tablets, which are sitting in a pill-box in his bedside vanity. Between not sleeping well and missing his medication, Danny is convinced he will have a convulsion. He asks his doctor to check his level.

The next morning, the divalproex sodium level comes back 30 µg/ml. His doctor suggests that they load him with intravenous medication (Depacon), and then continue his medications IV. Danny weighs 150 pounds, or 68.2 kg.

The formula for valproate loading is the same as for phenytoin, but the Vd (Volume of distribution) changes. The Vd for valproate is approximately 0.2 L/kg. To calculate the dose needed to bring Danny's level back to 70 µg/ml, we can use the formula:

$$\text{Dose} = \text{Weight (kg)} \times \text{Vd L/kg (desired level-current level)}$$

Dose = 68.2 kg × 0.2 L/kg (70µg/ml - 30 µg/ml)
Dose = 13.64 L × (40 µg/ml)
Dose = 545.6 mg

Danny receives a supplementary dose of 500 mg followed by IV Depacon 250 mg every six hours. The next morning his level is 63 µg/ml. He begins taking liquids two days later. The doctor discontinues Depacon and Danny returns to his usual dose of divalproex sodium tablets.

Resource K

Nonantiepileptic Drugs That Affect Phenytoin and Carbamazepine Levels

Increase Phenytoin Levels	Decrease Phenytoin Levels
Amiodarone	Folic acid
Azapropazone	Salicylates
Cimetidine	Tolbutamide
Chloramphenicol	Rifampin
Cotrimoxazole	Valproic acid
Dextropropoxyphene	
Diazepam	
Disulfiram	
Felbamate	
Fluconazole	
Fluoxetine	
Imipramine	
Metronidazole	
Miconazole	
Omeprazole	
Phenylbutazone	
Stiripentol	
Sulfaphenazole	
Isoniazid	
Increase Carbamazepine Levels	Decrease Carbamazepine Levels
Acetazolamide	Felbamate
Cimetidine	Phenobarbital
Clarithromycin	Phenytoin
Danazol	Primidone
Diltiazem	
Erythromycin	
Fluoxetine	
Isoniazid	
Propoxyphene	
Verapamil	

Resource L

Notes on Epilepsy Drugs for the Elderly

Carbamazepine (Tegretol)
- watch for hyponatremia, monitor serum sodium levels
- avoid cimetidine, erythromycin, and propoxyphene (these drugs will increase carbamazepine levels)
- may cause cardiac conduction defects and arrhythmias
- consider using slow-release forms (Carbatrol and Tegretol XR)

Felbamate (Felbatol)
- rarely necessary in elderly

Gabapentin (Neurontin)
- easiest drug to use in elderly, no drug interactions
- adjust dose for renal insufficiency

Lamotrigine (Lamictal)
- need lower dose when used with valproic acid
- risk of rash

Levetiracetam (Keppra)
- no drug interactions
- adjust dose for renal insufficiency

Oxcarbazepine (Trileptal)
- adjust dose for renal insufficiency
- watch for hyponatremia, monitor serum sodium levels
- *not* affected by cimetidine, erythromycin, or propoxyphene

Phenobarbital
- likely to cause confusion

Phenytoin (Dilantin)
- use lower doses, 200 mg/day may be sufficient
- can block cardiac conduction, consider alternatives in patients with heart block

Tiagabine (Gabitril)
- level drops when used with carbamazepine or phenytoin

Topiramate (Topamax)
- use low doses and titrate slowly to avoid cognitive symptoms
- use one half the usual dose in patients with moderate–severe renal impairment

Valproate (Depakote)
- use lower doses
- elevates lamotrigine level

- elevates carbamazepine epoxide level
- may increase tremor
- measure platelet count for patients on anticoagulation

Resource M

Pharmaceutical and Medical Device Companies: Medications, Web Sites, and Contact Information

- Abbott Laboratories (Depacon, Depakote, Tranzene, Tiagabine)
  http://www.abbott.com, (800) 222-6883
- Elan Pharmaceuticals (Diastat, Mysoline)
  http://www.athenaneuro.com, (650) 877-0900
- Cyberonics, Inc. (Vagal Nerve Stimulator)
  http://www.cyberonics.com, (800) 332-1375
- GlaxoWellcome (Lamictal)
  http://www.glaxowellcome.com, (800) 722-9292
- Novartis (Tegretol, Trileptal)
  http://www.novartis.com, (888) 644-8585
- Ortho-McNeil Pharmaceuticals (Topamax),
  http://www.ortho-mcneil.com, (800) 682-6532
- Parke-Davis (Celontin, Cerebyx, Dilantin, Neurontin, Zarontin)
  http://www.parke-davis.com/version_4/index.html, (800) 223-0432
- Roche Laboratories (Klonopin)
  http://www.roche.com, (800) 526-6367
- Sanofi Winthrop (Mebarol), (800) 446-6267
- Shire Richwood Pharmaceutical Group (Carbatrol) (800) 536-7878
- UCB Pharma (Keppra), (800) 477-7877
- Wallace Laboratories (Felbatol), (609) 655-6000
- Wyeth-Ayerst Lederle (Diamox, Phenobarbital)
  http://www.gwschamber.org.au/html/.wyeth-ayerst.html,
  (800) 934-5556

Resource N

Directory of Prescription Drug Patient Assistance Programs

Abbott (Depakote, Gabitril)
200 Abbott Park Road
D31C Building J23
Abbott Park, IL 60064
(800) 222-6885

Elan Pharmaceuticals (Diastat, Mysoline)
800 Gateway Blvd.
S. San Francisco, CA 94080
(800) 528-4362

GlaxoWellcome (Lamictal)
Box 52185
Phoenix, AZ 85072-9711
(800) 722-9294

Novartis (Tegretol, Tegretol-XR)
Box 52052
Phoenix, AZ 85072-9170
(800) 257-3273

Ortho-McNeil (Topamax)
Box 938
Somerville, NJ 08876
(800) 797-7737

Parke-Davis (Dilantin, Neurontin, Zarontin)
Box 1058
Somerville, NJ 08876
(908) 724-1247

Roche (Klonopin)
340 Kingsland Street
Nutley, NJ 07110
(800) 526-6367

Shire Richwood Pharmaceutical Group (Carbatrol)
7900 Tanners Gate Drive
Suite 200
Florence, KY 41042
(800) 536-7878

Wallace Laboratories (Felbatol)
Box 1001
Cranbury, NJ 08512
(800) 678-4657

Wyeth-Ayerst Lederle (Diamox)
Box 13806
Philadelphia, PA 19101
(800) 568-9938

Resource O

Internet Resources

Web Sites for Physicians

1. Antiepileptic Drug Pregnancy Registry
   http://neuro-www2.mgh.harvard.edu/aed/

2. American Academy of Neurology
   http://www.aan.com

3. American Epilepsy Association
   http://www.aesnet.org

4. Doctor's Guide to the Internet
   http://www.pslgroup.com/docguide.htm

5. Epilepsy Foundation
   http://www.efa.org

6. Epilepsy Information and Referral Services
   http://www.efa.org/what/info/index.htm

7. Epilepsy International.com
   http://epilepsy-international.com/english/

8. Epilepsy Links and Resources
   http://www.neuro.wustl.edu/epilepsy/linkresources.html

9. Epilepsy Ontario
   http://epilepsyontario.org/

10. National Institutes of Health
    http://www.ninds.nih.gov

11. Physician's Medical Law Letter
    http://www.mll.net

12. The Comprehensive Epilepsy Center
    http://neuro.med.cornell.edu/NYH-CMC/res19a.html

13. The Epilepsy Education Association, Inc.
    http://www.iupui.edu/~epilepsy/

14. Washington University Comprehensive Epilepsy Program
    http://www.neuro.wustl.edu/epilepsy

15. Woman and Epilepsy Initiative
    http://www.efa.org/what/wei/wei.html

16. YPWCnet Epilepsy Info Source
    http://www.ypwcnet.org/resource/epilep.htm

Resource P

Internet Resources

Web Sites for Patients

1. American Academy of Neurology Health and Wellness Information
   http://www.aan.com/neurovista

2. American Medical Women's Association
   http://www.amwa-doc.org

3. Epilepsy Foundation
   http://www.efa.org

4. Epilepsy-International.com
   http://www.epilepsy-international.com/english/index.html

5. Massachusetts General Hospital/Harvard Guide to Organizations
   Providing Epilepsy Support and Education
   http://neurosurgery.mgh.harvard.edu/ep-resrc.htm

6. Mike Chee's Epilepsy Home Page
   http://home.earthlink.net/~mchee1/gnrchm2.html

7. National Institutes of Health, Women's Health Initiative
   http://www.healthtouch.com

8. Sarah Pleasant's Epilepsy Resources
   http://www.geocities.com/hotsprings/2836/epilepsy.html

9. Stanford Comprehensive Epilepsy Center
   http://www.NeuroCentral.org

10. The Global Tuberous Sclerosis Information Link
    http://members.aol.com/gtsil/ts/index.htm

11. University of Florida
    http://www.vetmed.ufl.edu/ufmrg/dog

12. Washington University Comprehensive Epilepsy Program
    http://neuro.wustl.edu/epilepsy

Resource Q

National Association of Comprehensive Epilepsy Centers Directory
NAEC Facility Members and Program Directors as of May 1998

University of Alabama at Birmingham
Epilepsy Center—UAB
619 South 19th Street
Birmingham, AL 35233
Ruben Kuzniecky, MD
(205) 934-3866

Arkansas Comprehensive Epilepsy Program
800 Marshall Street
Little Rock, AR 72202-3591
Rick Boop, MD
(501) 320-1448

Arizona Comprehensive Epilepsy Program
UMC, Room 7303
1501 North Campbell
Tucson, AZ 85724
David Labiner, MD
(602) 694-6900

Barrow Neurological Institute Epilepsy Center
St. Joseph's Hospital and Medical Center
350 W. Thomas Road
Phoenix, AZ 85013-4496
Robert Fisher, MD, PhD
(602) 285-3390

Baylor College of Medicine
Epilepsy Center, The Methodist Hospital
Neurophysiology Department
6565 Fannin, MS M587
Houston, TX 77030
Peter Kellaway, MD
(713) 790-3109

Beth Israel Hospital
Comprehensive Epilepsy Center
330 Brookline Avenue
Boston, MA 02215
Donald Schomer, MD
(617) 667-3999

University of California at San Diego Epilepsy Center
200 W. Arbor Drive
San Diego, CA 92103
Vincent Iragui, MD, PhD
(619) 543-5302

University of California at San Francisco Epilepsy Center
400 Parnassus Avenue
Room 889, Box 1038
San Francisco, CA 94143
Kenneth Laxer, MD
(415) 476-6337

The Carolinas Epilepsy Center
Carolinas Medical Center
PO Box 32861
Charlotte, NC 28232
Steven Karner, MD
(704) 355-3949

Cedars-Sinai Medical Center
Division of Neurology
Room 8911, South Tower
8700 Beverly Boulevard
Los Angeles, CA 90048
Michel Levesque, MD
(310) 659-7475

Central Pennsylvania NeuroCenter
Comprehensive Epilepsy Center
2100 Harrisburg Pike
PO Box 3200
Lancaster, PA 17604-3200
Lawrence Rodichok, MD
(717) 290-3170

University of Chicago Hospital
Clinical Neurophysiology Labs
Room B206, Box 237
5841 South Maryland Avenue
Chicago, IL 60637
Jean-Paul Spire, MD
(312) 702-1780

Cleveland Clinic Foundation
Department of Neurology
9500 Euclid Avenue
Cleveland, OH 44106
Hans Lüders, MD
(216) 444-2200

CNI Epilepsy Center
Colorado Neurological Institute
701 E. Hampden, Suite 530
Englewood, CO 80110
Ronald E. Kramer, MD
(303) 788-4600

Columbia Comprehensive Epilepsy Center
The Neurological Institute
710 West 168th Street
New York, NY 10032
Timothy A. Pedley, MD
(212) 305-6489

Comprehensive Epilepsy Care Center for Children and Adults, PC
St. Lukes North Medical Building
222 South Woods Mill Road, Suite 610
Chesterfield, MO 63017
William E. Rosenfeld, MD
(314) 453-9300

Comprehensive Epilepsy Center
Allegheny General Hospital
320 East North Avenue
Pittsburgh, PA 15212
James P. Valeriano, MD
(412) 321-2162

Comprehensive Epilepsy Center for Children
Children's Hospital of Los Angeles
4560 Sunset Boulevard
Los Angeles, CA 90027
Interim Director
(213) 669-2498

Comprehensive Epilepsy Program
Sentara Norfolk General Hospital
600 Gresham Drive
Norfolk, VA 23507
Joseph Hogan, MD
(757) 668-3127

Comprehensive Epilepsy Program
Department of Neurology, Box BRH-E
University of Virginia Health Sciences Center
Charlottesville, VA 22908
Nathan B. Fountain, MD
(804) 243-6281

Duke Epilepsy Center
Box 2905
Duke University Medical Center
Durham, NC 27710
Rodney Radtke, MD
(919) 681-3448

Emory Epilepsy Center
Woodruff Memorial Building
Suite 6000, PO Drawer V
1639 Pierce Drive
Atlanta, GA 30322
Thomas R. Henry, MD
(404) 727-4887

Epilepsy Center of West Alabama
535 River Road East, Suite J2
Tuscaloosa, AL 35404
Alexandre B. Todorov, MD
(205) 553-4684

Epilepsy Monitoring Unit
Bowman Gray/Baptist Hospital Medical Center
Medical Center Boulevard
Winston-Salem, NC 27157
William L. Bell, MD
(919) 716-5281/extension 2317

The Epilepsy and Brain Mapping Program
10 Congress Street, Suite 505
Pasadena, CA 90017-4808
William W. Sutherling, MD
(626) 792-7300

Fairfax Hospital Neurodiagnostic Lab
3300 Gallows Road
Falls Church, VA 22046
James P. Simsarian, MD
(703) 698-3451

Medical College of Georgia
Department of Neurology
1459 Laney Walker Boulevard
Augusta, GA 30912
Donald W. King, MD
(404) 721-3325

Jefferson Comprehensive Epilepsy Center
111 South 11th Street, Suite 4150
Philadelphia, PA 19107
Michael Sperling, MD
(215) 955-1222

Henry Ford Hospital
Comprehensive Epilepsy Program
2799 W. Grand Boulevard
Detroit, MI 48202
Gregory L. Barkley, MD
(313) 876-3922

Immanuel Medical Center
6901 No. 72nd Street
Omaha, NE 68122
Richard Andrews, MD
(402) 572-2566

Indiana University Comprehensive Epilepsy Program
Riley Hospital, Room 5999C
702 Barnhill Drive
Indianapolis, IN 46202-5200
Omkar N. Martkland, MD
(317) 274-0181

Long Island Jewish Medical Center
Department of Neurology
Room 222
New Hyde Park, NY 11042
Neil Schaul, MD
(718) 470-7312

Marshfield Epilepsy Program
Department of Neurosciences
1000 North Oaks Avenue
Marshfield, WI 54449-5777
Kevin H. Ruggles, MD
(715) 387-5998

Maryland Epilepsy Center
Department of Neurology
22 South Greene Street
Baltimore, MD 21201-1595
Gregory K. Bergey, MD
(401) 328-6484

Miami Children's Hospital
Comprehensive Epilepsy Center
6125 SW 31st Street
Miami, FL 33155
Michael S. Duchowny, MD
(305) 662-8330

Medical City Dallas Hospital
7777 Forest Lane
Dallas, TX 75320
Richard North, MD
(214) 661-7684

University of Michigan Epilepsy Program
Department of Neurology
IB/0036 U. Hospital
Ann Arbor, MI 48109-0036
Ivo J. Drury, MD
(313) 936-9070

MINCEP Epilepsy Care
5775 Wayzata Boulevard
Minneapolis, MN 55416
Robert J. Gumnit, MD
(612) 525-2400

Minnesota Epilepsy Group
United Hospital
310 N. Smith Avenue, Suite 300
St. Paul, MN 55102
John R. Gates, MD
(612) 220-5290

Medical College of Ohio
Comprehensive Epilepsy Center
3000 Arlington Avenue
Toledo, OH 43699-0008
Thomas Swanson, MD
(419) 381-3544

NYU–HJD Comprehensive Epilepsy Center
Hospital for Joint Diseases
301 East 17th Street
New York, NY 10003
Orrin Devinsky, MD
(212) 598-6512

University of North Carolina
Department of Neurology
738 Burnett Womack building
Chapel Hill, NC 27514
John A. Messenheimer, MD
(919) 966-3707

Northwestern Memorial Hospital
Neurology Testing Center, 10th Floor
Passavant Pavilion
303 E. Superior
Chicago, IL 60611
Albert Ehle, MD
(312) 980-0484

Norwalk Hospital
Section of Neurology
Department of Medicine
Maple Street
Norwalk, CT 06851
Steven A. Jerrett, MD
(203) 852-2400

Comprehensive Oklahoma Program for Epilepsy
Department of Neurology
PO Box 26901—Room 3SP203
920 Stanton L. Young Boulevard
Oklahoma City, OK 73190
Kalarickal Oommen, MD
(405) 271-4113

Reed Neuro Research Center
UCLA School of Medicine
710 Westwood Plaza
Los Angeles, CA 90024
Jerome Engel Jr., MD
(310) 825-5745

University of Rochester Medical Center
Comprehensive Epilepsy Program
601 Elmwood Avenue, Box 673
Rochester, NY 14620-8673
Giuseppe Erba, MD
(716) 275-0698

Roper Hospital Epilepsy Program
Epilepsy Unit—5 West
316 Calhoun Street
Charleston, SC 29401
Alton Bryant, MD
(803) 723-0202

Rush Epilepsy Center
1653 West Congress Parkway
Chicago, IL 60612
Michael C. Smith, MD
(312) 942-5939

St. Francis Regional Medical Center
Epilepsy Center
929 North St. Francis
Wichita, KS 67214
William B. Svoboda, MD
(316) 268-8500

Sacramento Comprehensive Epilepsy Program
1020 29th Street, Suite 360
Sacramento, CA 95816
Robert S. Burgerman, MD
(910) 733-8915

Sacred Heart Regional Epilepsy Center
421 Chew Street
Allentown, PA 18102
Rajesh Sachdeo, MD
(215) 776-5166

Stanford Comprehensive Epilepsy Center
Department of Neurology, H3160
Stanford University Medical Center
Stanford, CA 94305
Martha Morrell, MD
(415) 725-6648

Swedish Medical Center
801 Broadway, Suite 830
Seattle, WA 98122
Allen Wyler, MD
(206) 386-3880

University of Texas Southwestern Epilepsy Center
Parkland Health and Hospital System
5201 Harry Hines Boulevard
Dallas, TX 75235
Paul Van Ness, MD
(214) 648-9356

Virginia Commonwealth
Medical College of Virginia
Department of Neurology
Box 559, MCV Station
Richmond, VA 23298-0599
R. J. DeLorenzo, MD, PhD
(804) 786-9720

Washington University Epilepsy Program
Department of Neurology and Neurological Surgery
Box 8111
660 South Euclid Avenue
St. Louis, MO 63110
John W. Miller, MD
(314) 362-7177

Resource R

Checklist for Women and Pregnancy

Preconception

- Does the woman have epilepsy?
- Is she taking the minimal number of antiepileptic drugs (AEDs) necessary to control her seizures?
- Is she taking the minimal doses of the AEDs necessary to control her seizures?
- Has she had a recent AED level?
- Is she taking folate at least 1 mg/day?
- If she has a personal or family history of fetal malformations, or is taking carbamazepine or valproate, is she taking folate 4 mg/day?
- Is she taking a prenatal vitamin?
- Does she have a genetic epilepsy syndrome?
- Has she had genetic counseling?
- Has she had epilepsy education?
- Is she taking an enzyme-inducing AED (barbiturate, carbamazepine, oxcarbazepine, phenytoin, or topiramate), which can interfere with the birth control pill or levonorgestrel implants (Norplant)?
- Has she had trouble with conception?
- Does she have prolonged menstrual bleeding (> 7days)?
- Does she have a menstrual cycle that is too short (< 21 days) or too long (> 35 days)?
- Is there evidence of polycystic ovary syndrome (polycystic ovaries, hirsutism, acne, obesity, elevated androgens, an elevated LH:FSH ratio, chronic anovulation, and insulin resistance)?
- Does she need referral to a gynecologist or endocrinologist?

Postconception

- Has she contacted the AED pregnancy registry (888) 233-2334?
- Has she informed her obstetrician of her pregnancy and seizure disorder?
- Has she had a serum alpha-fetoprotein level at 14–16 weeks?
- Has she had a level II (structural) ultrasound at 16–20 weeks gestation?
- Is amniocentesis at 16–20 weeks for alpha-fetoprotein and acetylcholinesterase levels necessary?
- Has she received oral Vitamin K1 10 mg/day, beginning at 36 weeks?
- Has she had a recent serum AED level checked?
- Has she learned safe ways of bathing and dressing the baby?

Postpartum

- Has the infant received 1 mg of Vitamin K1?
- Has the mother had an AED level checked and AED dosage reduced if needed?
- Is the baby sedated from breast-feeding?
- Is the mother getting enough rest?
- Is she using appropriate contraception?
- Has the infant had a normal examination by a pediatrician?

Resource S

Generalized Convulsive Status Epilepticus Protocol*

Minutes 0–5

- Evaluate airway and cardiorespiratory function, administer oxygen by cannula or mask, assess need for intubation and ventilatory assistance, attach oximeter
- History and focused examination: vital signs, level of consciousness, focal findings, seizure type
- Draw laboratories: antiepileptic drug (AED) blood levels, arterial blood gas, glucose, calcium, magnesium, electrolytes, complete blood count, prothrombin and partial thromboplastin time, toxic screen, blood and urine cultures
- Insert intravenous (IV) line, run 0.9 percent saline and 100 mg of thiamine IV
- If hypoglycemic or glucose level not back, give 50 ml IV bolus of 50 percent glucose, (children 25 percent glucose at 2 ml/kg)
- Record electrocardiogram

Minutes 5–20

- Diazepam 5 mg/min IV up to 20 mg. Anticipate respiratory depression. (Or lorazepam, 2 mg/min up to 4 mg)
- Load with phenytoin 20 mg/kg at up to 50 mg/min, monitor EKG and blood pressure, (reduce rate to 25 mg/min in elderly)
- Or, load with fosphenytoin, same dose in phenytoin equivalents (PE), can give at 150 PE/min

Minutes 20–40

- If patient still seizing, transfer to intensive care unit
- Draw phenytoin level
- Administer additional phenytoin or fosphenytoin at 5mg/kg until 30 mg/kg reached
- Administer phenobarbital 20 mg/kg IV at 60 mg/min
- Intubate and ventilate, if not already doing so

Minutes 40+

- Anesthesia protocol with pentobarbital, midazolam, or propofol

Pentobarbital

- 10–15 mg/kg at 50 mg/min IV, then 0.5–1 mg/kg/hr infusion. Titrate to burst suppression pattern on electroencephalogram (EEG). Bursts should last 1–2 seconds, suppression 5–10 seconds
- Draw pentobarbital level, initial goal 10–20 µg/ml
- Manage hypotension by decreasing pentobarbital dose, fluid bolus, or dopamine

Midazolam

- 0.2 mg/kg slow bolus and infuse 0.75–10 µg/kg/min

Propofol

- 1-2 mg/kg and continue at 2–10 mg/kg/hr

Then:

- Computed axial tomography brain scan or magnetic resonance imaging
- Consider lumbar puncture
- Continue maintenance AEDs and follow levels
- Daily EEG

---

*This protocol originates from the consensus conference of 1/17/98, published in *Neurology* 1998, Vol 51, #5, Supplement 4, with minor modifications from my own experience. There are many variations on this theme. Some physicians prefer lorazepam to diazepam because of its longer half-life. Others prefer a midazolam rather than pentobarbital drip. Thiopental anesthesia also has been used. A patient's allergies also influence medication choice. The value of a familiar protocol is to allow quick and correct implementation without losing time searching for the nearest *Washington Manual*. Therapy for convulsive status epilepticus should be aggressive and rapid and is best carried out by an experienced team.

Resource T
Home Safety Checklist

- Take precautions against burns! Avoid a gas stove and cook with an electric or microwave oven.
- Use rear burners when cooking.
- Use oven mitts.
- Use cart for hot food to wheel to table from stove.
- Install heat control devices in kitchen faucet and bathroom to prevent scalding.
- Carpet all floors.
- Use plastic containers rather than glass.
- Do not lock bathroom door.
- Take bath with only a few inches of water.
- Use handheld shower head and sit during shower.
- Choose a one floor dwelling if possible; limit stairs.
- Use an iron which shuts off automatically.
- Avoid using a curling iron.
- Keep a protective screen in front of the fireplace.
- Avoid exposed heaters.
- Do not smoke cigarettes.
- Install smoke alarms.
- Check in with a friend or family member at least once a day.
- Keep doctor's number by telephone.
- Make sure friend or family member has doctor's number.
- Instruct friends and family on proper first aid for convulsions and when to call an ambulance.
- Consider home security system with "panic button."

Resource U

The 10 Most Relevant Treatment Errors in Epilepsy[1]

1. **Failure to ensure the maximum tolerated dose in uncontrolled epilepsy.** Patients often are switched to another antiepileptic drug (AED) following a "breakthrough" seizure because their drug level is within the "therapeutic range." Rather than abandon a drug at a certain laboratory value, it can be more effective to increase dosage until toxic symptoms develop or seizures are controlled. (One might argue that when seizures continue, the drug is *not* within the "therapeutic range" for that patient.) In one study, almost one third of uncontrolled patients became seizure-free at a higher AED dose.

2. **Adding a second drug before the original one has failed.** In most cases, the toxicity of two or more drugs outweighs the potential therapeutic benefit of combination therapy. Patients often have toxic symptoms related to polypharmacy and unfavorable drug-drug interactions without much improvement in seizure control. Approximately 70 percent of patients can be controlled with monotherapy. Two or three drugs will lead to seizure control in another 15 percent to 20 percent.

   Three drugs rarely benefit a patient more than two drugs. Try monotherapy with at least three first-line AEDs before prescribing combination therapy.

3. **Delayed referral to specialized epilepsy units.** There are now epilepsy centers in more than half the states in the United States and in many foreign countries. These centers provide comprehensive care for patients with difficult-to-control seizures and are an excellent resource for management or a second opinion. A comprehensive epilepsy center offers psychosocial support, drug trials, surgery evaluation, and other therapies, such as the ketogenic diet and the vagal nerve stimulator. For patients who are good candidates, epilepsy surgery can produce miraculous results and should be done sooner rather than later. (See Resource Q.)

---

[1]Schmidt, D. *Epilepsia*, Suppl. 6, 1998, Vol. 39, p. 195.

4. **Misdiagnosis of frontal lobe seizures as nonepileptic psychogenic seizures.** Frontal lobe epileptic seizures may clinically simulate pseudoseizures, with thrashing movements, elaborate automatisms, and an absent or minimal postictal state. In addition, epileptic discharges may not appear on the scalp electroencephalogram (EEG). An experienced epileptologist relies on history, neurologic exam, video-EEG, neuroimaging, and neuropsychological evaluation to make the diagnosis.

5. **Failure to diagnose the epilepsy syndrome.** Accurate diagnosis of the epilepsy syndrome, such as benign rolandic epilepsy in children, allows one to reassure parents that the epilepsy is age-related and will disappear in adolescence. On the other hand, recognition of myoclonic epilepsy of Janz identifies a genetic epilepsy likely to be lifelong and strongly supports valproate as the preferred treatment. Failure to accurately diagnose epilepsy syndromes leads to less than optimal medication selection and clumsy medical management.

6. **Suboptimal use of new antiepileptic drugs.** Seven new AEDs have been approved by the Food and Drug Administration since 1993. Some patients who have failed conventional therapy show significant improvement with these new drugs. For example, at least 5 percent of patients started on topiramate become seizure-free. Most of the new drugs require careful titration and knowledge of drug interactions, but they should not be overlooked in the treatment of the intractable epilepsy patient.

7. **Unnecessary high dose of antiepileptic drugs.** Side effects must often be balanced against seizure control. High doses with clinical toxicity may not improve seizure control and, paradoxically, may even increase seizure frequency.

   Side effects occur in more than 50 percent of patients treated with AEDs. Patients may find these symptoms less acceptable than seizures. Compliance deteriorates when patients experience toxicity.

8. **Failure to use the optimum drug for seizure type.** Carbamazepine and phenytoin can worsen absence, atonic, and myoclonic seizures. Gabapentin also may exacerbate myoclonic jerks. On the other hand, valproate can be very effective for myoclonic seizures. A directed history or video-EEG can often clarify a patient's symptoms and lead to more effective therapy.

9. **Premature or impatient discontinuation of anticonvulsants in seizure-free patients.** Although many children succeed in "outgrowing" their seizures, this phenomenon is less common in

adults. Publications on seizure recurrence are of limited value in clinical practice because of the heterogeneity of study patients. Extrapolating statistical results to a specific patient can be difficult. The history, neurologic examination, EEG, and neuroimaging results can provide a guideline regarding the likelihood of seizures after AED withdrawal (see Chapter 3). If all of these factors are normal, the patient is likely to do well. If not, there is a significant risk of seizure recurrence.

10. **Failure to persistently pursue treatment goals.** It would seem to go without saying that all epilepsy patients want to be seizure-free. Yet, many patients and physicians accept small numbers of seizures per month or year as inevitable. Although infrequent, these seizures disrupt work, hinder social interaction, and create anxiety. Many of these patients remain on static, ineffective medication regimens. With the multitude of treatment options now available, every doctor visit becomes an opportunity to maximize therapy and work toward the goal of seizure freedom. Although there are patients who are refractory to therapy, their number shrinks daily.

Resource V

Compliance

Noncompliance with antiepileptic drugs (AEDs) is a widespread problem that has significant consequences. Twenty-five percent of cases of status epilepticus result from noncompliance. Fifty percent of "breakthrough" seizures that send patients to the emergency room are related to noncompliance. Unexplained variability in AED levels is usually the result of noncompliance.

The medical and social costs of AED noncompliance are high. Patients may lose a driver's license or job because of medication noncompliance.

Because noncompliance hinders care in as many as 50 percent of epilepsy patients, addressing compliance issues in an office visit can yield important long-term benefits. The cause is not always the same for each patient. Here is a summary of reasons for noncompliance, assessment techniques, and recommendations for improving patient compliance with AED therapy.

Reasons for Noncompliance

- Patient doesn't believe medication necessary (denial)
- Patient doesn't believe medication is helping
- Patient can't remember to take medication
- Medication is unwelcome reminder of epilepsy
- Medication causes side effects
- Irrational fear of medicine (friend died while taking medication)
- Rational fear of medicine (birth defects)
- Cost
- Inconvenience (midday dose)
- Regimen too complicated
- Multiple pharmacies
- Multiple prescribing physicians
- Alcohol and substance abuse
- Lack of reliable caregiver
- Chaotic life style

Assessing Compliance

- Patient interview
- Count pills
- Drug levels
- Electronic recording pill box
- Therapeutic effect

Recommendations to Improve Compliance

- Patient education
- Pill box (free)
- Seizure calendar (free)
- Physician samples (free)
- Indigent program for medications (see Resource N)
- More frequent physician visits (not free)
- Telephone reminders to patient
- Link medication taking to other activities; brushing teeth, meals, bedtime
- Drug level monitoring
- Successful seizure control

Resource W

First Aid for Seizures

Note: Most seizures are self-limited and require little intervention. Here are some practical guidelines.

Generalized Tonic Clonic Seizure

- Remain calm.
- Protect the patient from hurting himself/herself. Remove furniture and sharp objects from the area. Protect the patient's head by putting something soft—a pillow or folded clothing—beneath the head.
- Turn the patient on his/her side to prevent aspiration.
- Do not put anything in the patient's mouth.
- Do not restrain the patient's movements.
- Do not attempt cardiopulmonary resuscitation (CPR) unless the patient is clearly apneic.
- Time the seizure. Call for emergency services if jerking movements last longer than two minutes.
- Evaluate the patient for possible injuries sustained during seizure—concussion, fractures, lacerations. Send patient to emergency room if necessary.
- Stay with the patient until postictal confusion clears.
- Call for emergency services if postictal confusion lasts longer than 15 minutes. Patient may be having ongoing subclinical seizures.
- Notify patient's physician of seizure. Patient may need assessment for intercurrent illness, alcohol withdrawal, or substance abuse that may have triggered seizure.
- Do not allow patient to drive.
- Tell the patient what happened. Ask what he/she wants to do.

Partial Complex Seizure

- Do not restrain the patient.
- Protect the patient from wandering by gently guiding them into a safe area.
- Do not try to reason with patient during the seizure.
- Stay with the patient until confusion clears.
- Notify patient's physician of seizure.
- Do not allow the patient to drive.
- Tell the patient what happened. Ask what he/she wants to do.

If this is a first seizure, the patient requires immediate emergency room evaluation to rule out treatable causes for seizure such as meningitis, encephalitis, ruptured arteriovenous malformation, and brain tumor. A prompt informed decision must also be made regarding AED therapy.

Resource X
Safety Checklist for Procedures

Before Surgery

- Avoid sleep deprivation.
- Avoid elective surgery at time of month patient is likely to have seizures.
- Review medication allergies.
- Discuss patient history with anesthesiologist and surgeon regarding likelihood of perioperative seizure.
- Review seizure first aid with operative team, dentist, gynecologist, etc.
- Check serum antiepileptic drug (AED) levels before surgery.
- Optimize AED level with additional doses of medication if needed.
- Continue prescribed AEDs until just before surgery (if allowed).
- If prescribed AEDs cannot be given orally (because of gastrointestinal surgery or nausea and vomiting, for example) substitute with intravenous phenytoin or intravenous valproate (load intravenously using formula in Resource J).
- Check serum AED levels daily while patient in hospital.
- If patient taking valproate, check platelet count and bleeding time. If abnormal, consider lowering dose, changing to another AED, and postponing elective surgery.
- Avoid enflurane anesthesia; its isomer isoflurane is preferable.
- Ketamine hydrochloride may trigger seizures.

After surgery:

- Watch for drug interactions with pain medications.
- Check AED levels.
- Resume preoperative AEDs and dosing.

Resource Y

Driving and Epilepsy

State	Seizure-Free Period (months)*	Physician Must Report?
Alabama	6	No
Alaska	6	No
Arizona	3	No
Arkansas	12	No
California	3–12	Yes
Colorado	No set period	No
Connecticut	No set period	No
Delaware	No set period	Yes
District of Columbia	12	No
Florida	No set period	No
Georgia	12	No
Hawaii	12	No
Idaho	6	No
Illinois	No set period	No
Indiana	No set period	No
Iowa	6	No
Kansas	6	No
Kentucky	3	No
Louisiana	6	No
Maine	3	No
Maryland	3	No
Massachusetts	6	No
Michigan	6	No
Minnesota	6	No
Mississippi	12	No
Missouri	6	No

State	Seizure-Free Period (months)*	Physician Must Report?
Montana	No set period	No
Nebraska	3	No
Nevada	3	Yes
New Hampshire	12	No
New Jersey	12	Yes
New Mexico	12	No
New York	12	No
North Carolina	6–12	No
North Dakota	3–6	No
Ohio	No set period	No
Oklahoma	12	No
Oregon	6	Yes
Pennsylvania	6	Yes
Puerto Rico	24	No
Rhode Island	18	No
South Carolina	6	No
South Dakota	6–12	No
Tennessee	6	No
Texas	6	No
Utah	3	No
Vermont	No set period	No
Virginia	6	No
Washington	6	No
West Virginia	12	No
Wisconsin	3	No
Wyoming	3	No

*In many cases, these time frames are modifiable depending on a given patient's circumstances and a physician's recommendation. Information in this table updated as of September 1998.

Resource Z

A Short Course in Electroencephalography (EEG)

More so than many other diagnostic tests, interpretation formats and styles of EEG reports vary significantly from institution to institution and from reader to reader. Even the vocabulary chosen to describe and interpret certain findings defies standardization. One reader's "sharp wave" is another's "sharp transient." Consequently, the clinical implications of an EEG report are not always crystal clear.

State-dependent findings also complicate EEG interpretation. A slow wave during sleep may be normal, yet a wave of identical configuration and frequency occurring while awake indicates an underlying lesion. The definition of "normal" also varies with age. Infant EEGs differ dramatically from adult recordings.

This section highlights a few EEG basics as well as key words to look for in an EEG report that convey particular clinical significance. Examples of EEG jargon from actual reports appear below with explication.

A routine EEG consists of 20 minutes of brain waves. The results may be displayed digitally on a video screen or printed on approximately 120 pages of EEG paper. Ideally, a technician records samples of awake, drowsy, and sleep states during this period. (Some patients only have epileptic activity during sleep.)

A technician administers two provocative tests during a standard EEG, hyperventilation and photic stimulation. The patient is asked to hyperventilate for 3 to 5 minutes. This maneuver lowers intracerebral carbon dioxide levels and brings out epileptic and other abnormal activity. (Hyperventilation reveals epileptic activity in children with untreated absence seizures 80 percent of the time.)

Photic stimulation elicits epileptic activity in 5 percent of patients with epilepsy. Patients with primary generalized epilepsy rather than localization-related epilepsy (see Resource A) are much more likely to demonstrate this response. Occasionally, the strobe light triggers a convulsion.

In many normal patients, photic stimulation elicits a phenomenon known as "photic driving" at certain flash frequencies. During photic driving, the background EEG synchronizes with the strobe frequency.

Sleep deprivation the night before an EEG also acts as an activation procedure. In a patient with epilepsy, sleep deprivation increases the likelihood that epileptic discharges will appear on the recording.

Waves are described in terms of amplitude, morphology and frequency (cycles/second or Hertz). The most common waves are:

- Alpha (8–13 Hertz)
- Beta (> 13 Hertz)
- Theta (4–7 Hertz)
- Delta < 4 Hertz)

Alpha waves constitute the normal background in adults. Beta waves (see below) may be pathologic, but they shed little insight on whether a patient has epilepsy. Theta and delta waves are slow waves. They normally occur in drowsiness and sleep, but often are abnormal when seen in the awake state.

Examples from EEG reports:

Normal findings

The amplitudes of the awake background activities were low, ranging between 10 and 25 microvolts and the frequencies consisted largely of irregularly modulated very fast frequency beta activities appearing diffusely.

An EEG reader should always comment on the background, which often is composed of alpha and beta frequencies. "Background amplitude," unless distinctly asymmetric or exceptionally low, can largely be ignored. (Abnormalities of frequency are more common than amplitude.)

"Beta" waves indicate a fast frequency that may be due to drugs, such as barbiturates and benzodiazepines, or early alcohol withdrawal. "Beta" waves also occur in many normal people.

Intermittent photic stimulation produced well-defined bilaterally symmetric occipital driving responses.

A normal finding. See above.

With hyperventilation, some generalized slowing is appreciated toward the end of this procedure. This quickly dissipates after hyperventilation is terminated.

Generalized slowing commonly occurs with hyperventilation. When the slowing resolves promptly (within 30 seconds) after the discontinuation of hyperventilation, it is considered normal.

Abnormal findings

There was a lot of movement artifact associated with persistent leg and arm movement.

Artifacts are waveforms that do not originate in the brain. Because brain waves are of such low amplitude, electrical disturbances from the heart and other muscles, eye blinks, movement of electrodes, wires, and medical equipment can easily contaminate the EEG record. Many artifacts simulate epileptic and other pathologic activity. Artifacts must be recognized in order to properly interpret an EEG.

One must consider repeating the record when a large amount of artifact is present on an EEG, as true brain abnormalities may be obscured.

There is a mild, continuous, generalized, nonspecific disturbance of cerebral activity.

Hospitalized patients with a toxic-metabolic encephalopathy often have an EEG like this. As in electrocardiogram interpretation, the term *nonspecific* does not mean "unimportant." A nonspecific abnormality on the EEG indicates cerebral dysfunction that may be due to a wide variety of causes. In this case, because the abnormality is "generalized," an underlying focal lesion such as a tumor or hemorrhage is unlikely.

Definite left anterior temporal spikes occur intermittently. Phase reversal occurs at T3.

The presence of "spikes" usually indicates epilepsy. To be called a spike, a wave must fulfill certain strict criteria regarding duration, morphology, and context. When an electroencephalographer uses this term, the findings are unequivocal.

A "phase reversal" indicates the origin of the electrical discharge. "T" stands for temporal; "3" refers to the position on the lateral side of the head. (All odd numbers are on the left side of the head. Even numbers are on the right.) Consequently, this EEG description strongly suggests left temporal lobe epilepsy.

There are frequent episodes of sharp and slow waves and theta activity in the left temporal region.

The EEG reader has detected a focal abnormality. A temporal lobe sharp wave suggests epilepsy, but it is not as definitive as a spike. (Not all sharp waves, however, are pathologic.)

Theta waves are slow waves. Delta waves are slower and more significant.

A focal abnormality suggests an underlying lesion that may be structural. In general, patients with a focal EEG abnormality should be evaluated with computed axial tomography or magnetic resonance imaging to further evaluate the etiology of this finding.

If you are able to review several EEG reports with your electroencephalographer, you will gain a better appreciation for the meaning behind the words.

Resource AA

Heidelberg Declaration on Epilepsy

25 October 1998

At a meeting in Heidelberg, Germany, on 25 October 1998, over 100 leaders of European professional and lay bodies, World Health Organization representatives and health experts from governments and universities unanimously agreed on the following declaration:

- Six million people in Europe currently have epilepsy. Fifteen million will have epilepsy at some time in their lives
- Epilepsy has profound physical, psychological, and social consequences
- Children, adolescents, and the elderly are especially afflicted by non-detection and under-treatment
- With appropriate treatment over three quarters of people with epilepsy could lead normal lives free of seizures
- Epilepsy costs the countries of Europe over 20 billion ECU every year, an amount that could be significantly reduced with effective action

We call on the governments of Europe, the European Union, and all health care providers to join us in taking strong and decisive action to meet the objectives of the Global Campaign against Epilepsy launched by the World Health Organization, International League Against Epilepsy (ILAE), and International Bureau for Epilepsy (IBE). Specifically, we urge action:

- to improve public understanding of epilepsy and thereby reduce its stigma
- to remove discrimination against people with epilepsy in the workplace
- to help people with epilepsy to understand their condition and to empower them to seek appropriate treatment and lead fulfilled lives
- to improve the knowledge of health care professionals and other professionals about epilepsy, before and after graduation
- to ensure the availability of modern equipment, facilities, trained personnel and the full range of antiepileptic drugs, so that an accurate diagnosis can be made leading to the most effective treatment
- to encourage research on epilepsy and its management

- to encourage close liaison among governments, health and social authorities and agencies, and the national chapters of the ILAE and IBE
- to support the publication of a "white paper" as a detailed Public Health statement on Epilepsy in Europe
- to provide practical assistance for countries with underdeveloped epilepsy services within and beyond Europe

Resource AB

National and State Epilepsy Resources

Antiepileptic Drug Pregnancy Registry
149 CNY-MGH East, Room 5022A
Charlestown, MA 02129-2000
(888) 233-2334
(617) 724-8307 fax
aed.registry@helix.mgh.harvard.edu

American Epilepsy Society
American Branch International League Against Epilepsy
638 Prospect Avenue
Hartford, Connecticut 06105-4240
(860) 586-7505
(860) 586-7550 fax
info@aesnet.org

Epilepsy Foundation
4351 Garden City Drive
Landover, MD 20785
(800) EFA-1000
(301) 459-3700

Epilepsy Foundation Library
(800) 332-4050

State Epilepsy Foundation Affiliates

Alabama
Epilepsy Foundation of North and Central Alabama
1801 Oxmoor Road, Suite 101
Birmingham, AL 35209
(800) 950-6662

Epilepsy Chapter of Mobile and Gulf Coast
951 Government Street, Suite 201
Mobile, AL 36604
(334) 432-0970

Arizona
Epilepsy Foundation of Arizona
PO Box 25084
Phoenix, AZ 85002
(602) 406-3581

California
Epilepsy Foundation of Los Angeles and Orange Counties
3600 Wilshire Boulevard, Suite 920
Los Angeles, CA 90010
(213) 382-7337

Epilepsy Foundation of Northern California
1624 Franklin Street, Suite 900
Oakland, CA 94612
(510) 893-6272

Epilepsy Society of San Diego County
2055 El Cajon Boulevard
San Diego, CA 92104
(619) 296-0161

Colorado
Epilepsy Foundation of Colorado, Inc.
234 Columbine Street, Suite 333
Denver, CO 80206
(303) 377-9774

Connecticut
Epilepsy Foundation of Connecticut, Inc.
1800 Silas Deane Highway, #168
Rocky Hill, CT 06067
(860) 721-9226

Delaware
Epilepsy Foundation of Delaware
New Castle Corporate Commons
61 Corporate Circle
New Castle, DE 19720
(302) 324-4455

Florida
The Epilepsy Foundation of Northeast Florida, Inc.
6028 Chester Avenue, Room 106
Jacksonville, FL 32217
(904) 731-3752

Epilepsy Foundation of South Florida, Inc.
Chase Federal Building
7300 N. Kendall Drive, Suite 700
Miami, FL 33156
(305) 670-4949

Epilepsy Foundation of Southwest Florida, Inc.
1900 Main Street, Suite 212
Sarasota, FL 34236
(941) 953-5988

Epilepsy Foundation of Eastern Florida
5730 Corporate Way, Suite 220
West Palm Beach, FL 33407
(561) 478-6515

Georgia
Epilepsy Foundation of Georgia
100 Edgewood Ave, NE Suite 1200
Atlanta, GA 30303
(800) 527-7105

Hawaii
Epilepsy Foundation of Hawaii, Inc.
PO Box 61033
Honolulu, HI 96839
(808) 951-7705

Idaho
Epilepsy Foundation of Idaho
310 West Idaho
Boise, ID 83702
(800) 237-6676

Illinois
Epilepsy Foundation of Southwestern Illinois
1931 West Main Street
Belleville, IL 62226
(618) 236-2181

Epilepsy Foundation of Greater Chicago
20 E. Jackson Boulevard, 13th Floor
Chicago, IL 60611
(800) 273-6027

Epilepsy Foundation of Southern Illinois
1100 D South 42nd Street
Mt. Vernon, IL 62864
(618) 244-6680

Epilepsy Foundation of North/Central Illinois
321 West State Street, Suite 208
Rockford, IL 61101
(815) 964-2689

Louisiana
Epilepsy Foundation of SE Louisiana
3701 Canal Street, Suite I
New Orleans, LA 70119
(504) 486-6326

Massachusetts and Rhode Island
Epilepsy Foundation of Massachusetts and Rhode Island
95 Berkeley Street, Suite 409
Boston, MA 02116
(617) 542-2292

Maryland
Epilepsy Foundation of the Chesapeake Region
Hampton Plaza
300 E. Joppa Road, Suite 1103
Towson, MD 21286
(800) 492-2523

Michigan
Epilepsy Foundation of Michigan
26211 Central Park Boulevard, #100
Southfield, MI 48076
(800) 377-6226

Minnesota
Epilepsy Foundation of Lake Superior, Inc.
202A Ordean Building
424 West Superior Street
Duluth, MN 55802
(218) 726-4730

Epilepsy Foundation of Minnesota
2356 University Ave, W. #405
St. Paul, MN 55114
(612) 646-8675

Missouri
Epilepsy Foundation for the Heart of America Region
6550 Troost, Suite BC
Kansas City, MO 64131
(816) 444-2800

Epilepsy Foundation of the St. Louis Region
7100 Oakland Avenue
St. Louis, MO 63117
(314) 645-6969

Mississippi
Epilepsy Foundation of Mississippi
4795 McWillie Drive, Suite 101
Jackson, MS 39206
(601) 362-2761

North Carolina
Epilepsy Foundation of North Carolina, Inc.
3001 Spring Forest Road
Raleigh, NC 27616
(919) 876-7788

Nebraska and Iowa
Epilepsy Foundation of Nebraska and Iowa
6910 Pacific Street, Suite 103
Omaha, NE 68106
(402) 553-6567

New Jersey
Epilepsy Foundation of New Jersey
429 River View Plaza
Trenton, NJ 08611
(800) 336-5843

New York
Epilepsy Foundation of Northeastern New York
Three Washington Square
Albany, NY 12205
(518) 456-7501

The Epilepsy Foundation of Long Island, Inc.
550 Stewart Avenue
Garden City, NY 11530
(516) 794-5500

Epilepsy Foundation of New York City
305 7th Avenue, 12th Floor
New York, NY 10001
(212) 633-2930

Epilepsy Society of Southern New York, Inc.
1 Blue Hill Plaza, Box 1745
Pearl River, NY 10965
(914) 627-0627

Epilepsy Foundation of Rochester and Syracuse Regions
1000 Elmwood Avenue

Rochester, NY 14620
(800) 724-7930

Ohio
Epilepsy Council of Greater Cincinnati, Inc.
3 Centennial Plaza
895 Central Avenue
Cincinnati, OH 45202
(513) 721-2905

Epilepsy Foundation of Northeast Ohio
2800 Euclid Avenue, Room 450
Cleveland, OH 44115
(216) 579-1330

Epilepsy Foundation of Central Ohio
454 East Main Street, Suite 250
Columbus, OH 43215
(614) 228-4401

Epilepsy Foundation of Western Ohio
803 East 5th Street, Suite C
Dayton, OH 45402
(937) 222-0127

Oregon
Epilepsy Foundation of Oregon
619 SW 11th Avenue, Suite 225
Portland, OR 97205
(503) 228-7651

Pennsylvania
Epilepsy Foundation of Southeastern Pennsylvania
6th Floor Front
Seven Benjamin Franklin Pky
Philadelphia, PA 19103
(215) 523-9180

Epilepsy Foundation of Western Pennsylvania
Vocational Rehab Center
1323 Forbes Avenue, #102
Pittsburgh, PA 15219
(800) 361-5885

Puerto Rico
Soc Puertorriquena de Ayuda al Paciente con Epilepsia
Hospital Ruiz Soler

Calle Marginal Final
Bayamon, PR 00959
(787) 782-6200

South Carolina
Epilepsy Foundation of South Carolina
229 Parson Street
2nd Floor, Suite 5
West Columbia, SC 29169
(803) 926-0071

Tennessee
Epilepsy Foundation of Greater Chattanooga
744 McCallie Avenue, Suite 421
Chattanooga, TN 37403
(423) 756-1771

Epilepsy Foundation of Greater Knoxville
PO Box 3156
Knoxville, TN 37927
(423) 522-4991

Epilepsy Foundation of West Tennessee
4013 Premier Avenue
Memphis, TN 38118
(901) 795-6160

Epilepsy Foundation of Middle Tennessee
2002 Richard Jones Road, #C202
Nashville, TN 37215
(615) 269-7091

Texas
Epilepsy Foundation of Greater North Texas
2906 Swiss Avenue
Dallas, TX 75204
(214) 823-8809

Epilepsy Foundation of Southeast Texas
2650 Fountain View, Suite 316
Houston, TX 77057
(713) 789-6295

The Epilepsy Foundation of Central and South Texas
10615 Perrin Beitel, Suite 602
San Antonio, TX 78217
(210) 653-5353

Utah
Epilepsy Association of Utah

350 South 400 East, Suite 250
Salt Lake City, UT 84111
(801) 534-0210

Virginia
Epilepsy Association of Virginia
The Highlands Center
Box BRH-UVA Health Sciences Center
Charlottesville, VA 22908
(804) 924-8678

Vermont
Epilepsy Association of Vermont
BO Box 6292
Rutland, VT 05702
(802) 775-1686

Washington
Epilepsy Foundation Washington
3800 Aurora Avenue North, #370
Seattle, WA 98103
(206) 547-4551

Wisconsin
Epilepsy Foundation of Western Wisconsin
1812 Brackett Avenue, Suite 5
Eau Claire, WI 54701
(715) 834-4455

Epilepsy Association of Southern Wisconsin, Inc.
201 South Water Street
Janesville, WI 53545
(800) 693-2287

Epilepsy Center South Central
7617 Mineral Point Road
Madison, WI 53717
(800) 657-4929

Wisconsin Epilepsy Association
6400 Gisholt Drive, Suite 113
Madison, WI 53713
(800) 733-1244

Epilepsy Foundation of Southeast Wisconsin
735 North Water Street, Suite 701
Milwaukee, WI 53202
(414) 271-0110

Midstate Epilepsy Association

1004 First Street, Suite 5
Stevens Point, WI 54481
(800) 924-9932

Other
Epilepsy Information Service
Patricia Gibson, MSSW, Director
(800) 642-0500

Jim Abrahams, Director
The Charlie Foundation to Help Cure Pediatric Epilepsy
501 10th Street
Santa Monica, CA 90402
(information about ketogenic diet)

Keto Klub, Inc.
Elaine J. Huffman, President
61557 Miami Meadows Court
South Bend, IN 46614
(219) 299-3438
(information about ketogenic diet)

Resource AC
International Epilepsy Resources

International League Against Epilepsy (ILAE)
Epilepsie Zentrum Bethel
Mara 1 Maraweg 21
Bethel 33617
Bielefeld Germany
00 49 521 144 4897
00 49 521 144 4637 Fax

ILAE CHAPTERS as of March 1999

Algeria
Prof. Mahmoud Ait-Kaci-Ahmed
Vice-President, Algerian League against Epilepsy
Service de Neurologie
Hôpital Ali Ait-Idir
Boulevard A. Hahad
16000 Alger
Phone: +2132 96 33 28
Fax: +2132 96 38 25
E-mail maitkaci@hotmail.com

Argentina
Dr. Zenon M. Sfaello
Presidente
Liga Argentina contra la Epilepsia (LACE)
Boulevar Chacabuco 1068
Barrio Nueva Córdoba
5000 Córdoba
Phone: +5451 60 4101 or +5451 60 4250
Fax: +5451 60 8546

Secretariat
Liga Argentina contra la Epilepsia (L.A.C.E.)
a/c División Neurología
Sánchez de Bustamante 1399, p. 2E
1425 Buenos Aires
Phone/Fax: +541 962 4272 or +541 821 8581

Austria
Prof. Dr. Walter Stögmann
1. Vorsitzender, Österreichische Sektion der ILAE
Preyer'sches Kinderspital
Schrankenberggasse 31
A-1100 Wien
Phone: +431 60113 1301
Fax: +431 60113 1309

1st Secretary
Prof. Dr. Christoph Baumgartner
Universitätsklinik für Neurologie
Währinger Gürtel 18 - 20
A - 1090 Wien
Phone: +431 40400 3433
Fax: +431 40400 3141
E-mail   Christoph.Baumgartner@univie.ac.at

Australia
Dr. Andrew Black
President, Epilepsy Society of Australia
Department of Neurology
The Queen Elizabeth Hospital
28 Woodville Road
Woodville, SA 5011
Phone: +618 8222 6239
Fax: +618 8222 6093

Secretary
Dr. Christopher Rowe
Department of Neurology
The Queen Elizabeth Hospital
28 Woodville Road
Woodville, SA 5011
Phone: +618 8222 6239
Fax: +618 8222 6093

Brasil
Marilisa M. Guerreiro, M. D., Ph. D.
President
Liga Brasileira de Epilepsia
Rua Teodoro Sampaio, 741, Apto. 94
05405-050 São Paulo - SP -
Phone: +55 11 853 6574
Fax: +55 19 871 6715
E-mail guerreir@dglnet.com.br

Secretary
Maria Luiza G. de Manreza
Liga Brasileira de Epilepsia (LBE)
Rua Teodoro Sampaio 741, AptE 94
05405-050 São Paulo - SP -
Phone: +55 11 853 6574
Fax: +55 11 853 6574

Bulgaria
Prof. Dimitar Chavdarov
Bulgarian Association Against Epilepsy
Medical University, Dept. of Neurophysiology
1, G. Sofiiski str.
1431 Sofia
Phone: +3592 542941
Fax: +3592 525037
e-mail blae@medun.acad.bg

Burkina Faso
Dr. Kapouné Karfo
President
Ligue Burkinabe Contre l'Epilepsie (LBCE)
01 BP 2317, Ouagadougou 01
Province du Kadiogo

Canada
Richard S. McLachlan, M. D.
President, Canadian League Against Epilepsy
Dept. of Clinical Neurological Sciences
London Health Sciences Center
339 Windermere Road
London, Ontario N6A 5A5
Phone: +1 519 663 3341
Fax: +1 519 663 3753

Secretary-Treasurer
J. M. Dooley, M. D.
Neurology Division
IWK-Grace Health Centre
5850 University Avenue
HaliFax:, Nova Scotia, B3J 3G9
Phone: +1 902 428 8489
Fax: +1 902 428 8486
E-mail jdooley@is.dal.ca

Chile
Dr. Carlos Acevedo Schwartzmann
Presidente
Liga Chilena contra la Epilepsia
Cruz del Sur 133, of. 703
Santiago
Phone: +562 2085311 and +562 2085413
Fax: +562 699 4084
E-mail liche@entelchile.net

Secretary-General
Gabriela Saavedra Cruz
Erasmo Escala 2220
República
Santiago
Phone: +562 699 2288
Fax: +562 699 4084
E-mail liche@entelchile.net

Colombia
Dr. Jaime Fandiño Franky
Presidente, Liga Colombiana contra la Epilepsia
Cap. de Bolívar, Ternera, calle 1a., El Edén
Cartagena
Phone: +5756 618107 and +5756 618199
Fax: +5756 618111
E-mail fandino@cartagena.cetcol.net.co

Secretary:
Luis Enrique Morillo Zárate, M. D.
Liga Central contra la Epilepsia
Calle 35, NE 17-48
Bogotá
Phone: +5712 455717, 850788, and 877440

Democratic Republic of Congo
Prof. Kazadi Kayembe
Ligue Congolaise Contre l'Épilepsie
B.P. 825
Kinshasa XI

Secretary General
Dr, Mutombo Lukusa
Ligue Congolaise Contre l'Épilepsie
B.P. 825
Kinshasa XI

Republic of Croatia
Prof. Vera Dürrigl, M. D. Ph. D.
President
Croatian League against Epilepsy
Jurjevska 25
10000 Zagreb
Phone: +385 (0) 1 432 459
Fax: +385 (0) 1 425 173

Secretary General
Dr. Branka Marusi–Della Marina
Children's Hospital Zagreb
Zagreb University Medical School
Klaieva 16
10 000 Zagreb
Phone: +385 (0)1 44 04 55 or +3851 441 611
Fax: +385 (0)1 45 14 55

Cuba
Prof. Luis Rodríguez Rivera
Presidente, Liga Cubana contra la Epilepsia
Hospital Psiquiátrico de La Habana
Ave. Independencia No. 26520
Rpto. Mazorra Ap 9, Boyeros
C. Habana CP 19220
Phone: +537 451688, +537 451867, +537 411 519
Fax: +537 451512
E-mail sglezpal@infomed.sld.cu

Vicepresident - Secretary
Dr. Salvador Gonzaléz Pal
Hospital Psiquiátrico de La Habana
Ave. Independencia No. 26520
Rpto. Mazorra Ap 9, Boyeros
C. Habana CP 19220
Phone: +537 451688, +537 451867, +537 290041
Fax: +537 451512
E-mail sglezpal@infomed.sld.cu

Czech Republic
Pavel Mares, M. D. DSc.
President, Czech League against Epilepsy
Institute of Physiology, Academy of Sciences
Vídeská 1083
CZ - 14220 Prague 4
Phone: +4202 4751111
Fax: +4202 4752488
E-mail: marcsp@biomed.cas.cz

Vicepresident
Prof. Vladimír Komárek
Dept. of Child Neurology
Children Faculty Hospital
V úvalu 84 - Motol
CZ - 150 00 Prague 5
Phone: +4202 24 43 33 00
Fax: +4202 24 43 33 22
E-mail: vladimir.komarek@lfmotol.cuni.cz

Denmark
Dr. Jørgen Alving
President, Danish Epilepsy Society
Dianalund Epilepsy Hospital
Dept. of Neurophysiology
Kolonivej 1
DK - 4293 Dianalund
Phone: +4558 26 50 50 ext. 2449
Fax: +4558 26 44 61
E-mail kfjral@vestamt.dk

Secretary
Dr. Anne Sabers
Dianalund Epilepsy Hospital
Kolonivej 1
DK - 4293 Dianalund
Phone: +4558 265050, ext.2211
Fax: +4558 264315

Dominican Republic
Dr. Julio Oscar Tejada Jaquez
Tte. Amado Garcia Querrero No. 233
Santo Domingo

Ecuador
Dr. Jorge Pesantes
Presidente, Liga Ecuatoriana contra la Epilepsia
Italia 736 y Mariana de Jesús
P. O. Box 17-21-838
Quito
Phone: +5932 522109
Fax: +5932 569797

Secretary
Dr. Marcelo Placencia
Italia 736 y Mariana de Jesús
P. O. Box 17-21-838
Quito
Phone: +5932 522109
Fax: +5932 569797

Egypt
Prof. Dr. Farouk Koura
President, Egyptian Society against Epilepsy
Head of Neurology Department
Cairo University
13 Yossef El Gindy
Falaki Squ.
Cairo
Phone: +202 5852684

Secretary-General
Prof. Dr. Ahmed T. El-Ghonemy
Department of Neurology, Cairo University
32 Falaki Str.
Cairo
Phone: +202 34 803 88
Fax: +202 36 132 28

Finland
Prof. Mattii Sillanpää
President, Finnish Epilepsy Society
Department of Child Neurology
University of Turku Hospital TYKS
P. O. B. 21
SF - 20521 Turku
Phone: +358 22 61 2437
Fax: +358 22 61 1460
E-mail matti.sillanpaa@utu.fi

Secretary
Dr. Reetta Kälviäinen
Dept. of Neurology
University of Kuopio, University Hospital KYS
SF - 70211 Kuopio
Phone: +358 17 173 311
Fax: +358 17 173 031
E-mail reetta.kalviainen@kuh.fi

France
Dr. Charlotte Dravet
President, Ligue Française contre l'Épilepsie
Centre St. Paul
300, Bvd. Sainte Marguerite
F - 13009 Marseille
Phone: +334 91170750
Fax: +334 91 759669
E-mail csparep@infonie.fr

Secretary-General
Dr. Pierre Thomas
Service de Neurologie, Consultation d'Epileptologie
Hôpital Pasteur
30, Voie Romaine - B. P. 69
F - 06002 Nice cedex 1
Phone: +334 93819377
Fax: +334 93819377
E-mail piertho@calva.net

Germany
Prof. Dr. C. E. Elger
1. Vorsitzender, Deutsche Sektion der
Internationalen Liga gegen Epilepsie
Klinik für Epileptologie
Sigmund Freud-Str. 25
53105 Bonn
Phone: +49 228 2875727
Fax: +49 228 2874328
E-mail elger@mailer.meb.uni-bonn.de

Office
Geschäftsstelle der Deutschen Sektion
der Internationalen Liga gegen Epilepsie
Herforder Str. 5 - 7
D - 33602 Bielefeld
Phone: +49 521 12 41 92
Fax: +49 521 12 41 72
E-mail liga@ligaepilepsie.de

Georgia
Tina Geladze, M. D.
President, Georgian Society against Epilepsy
P. Saradgishivili Institute of Neurology
Epilepsy Research Center
Gudamakari 2
380092 Tbilisi
Phone: +995 32 618461
Fax: +995 32 001027
E-mail: david@gsae.org.ge

Secretary General
Nana Tatishvili, M. D.
P. Saradgishivili Institute of Neurology
Epilepsy Research Center
Gudamakari 2
380092 Tbilisi

Phone: +995 32 610448 or +995 320401
Fax: +995 32 227808
E-mail neuro@global-erty.net +
    david@gsae.org.ge

Great Britain
Dr. Tim A. Betts
President, British Branch of the ILAE
Queen Elizabeth Pschychiatric Hospital, Seizure Clinic
Mindlesohn Way
Edgbaston, Birmingham B15 2OZ
Phone: +44121 627 2852
Fax: +44121 627 2850
E-mail T.A.Betts@bham.ac.uk

Treasurer and Membership-Secretary
Dr. D. Fish
The National Society for Epilepsy
Chalfont St. Peter
Gerrards Cross
Buckinghamshire SL9 9RJ
Phone: +44 1494 601300
Fax: +44 1494 876 294

Greece
Prof. Aristides Kazis
President, Greek League against Epilepsy
Cr Neurologic Clinic
University of Thessaloniki
G. Papanicolaou Hospital
Thessaloniki
Phone: +3031 99 23 91
Fax: +3031 35 71 00

Secretary General
Dr. Ioannis Mavromatis
B Dept. of Neurology
University of Thessaloniki
AHEPA Hospital
Thessaloniki
Phone:+3031 99 46 76
Fax: +3031 20 43 68

Guatemala
Dr. Henry B. Stokes
Presidente, Capítulo Guatemala de la Liga
Internacional contra la Epilepsia CAGUALICE

6ª Calle 2 - 48 Zona 1
Guatemala
Phone:+5022 317858 or +5022 317866
Fax: +5022 514008
E-mail hstokes@infovia.com.gt

Office:
CAGUALICE, Capítulo Guatemala
Liga Internacional contra la Epilepsia
Av. La Reforma 1-64, zona 9
Guatemala
Phone: +502 2 317858 and +502 2 317866
Fax: +502 2 514008

Hungary
Dr. Péter Halász
President, Hungarian Chapter of the ILAE
Postgraduate Medical Univ., Dept. of Neurology
Hüvösvölgyi u. 116
H - 1021 Budapest
Phone: +361 391 5438
Fax: +361 391 5438
E-mail hal12197@helka.iif.hu or h12197hal@ella.hu

India
Dr. G. Arjundas
President, Indian Epilepsy Society
Mercury Nursing Home
36, Pantheon Road
Egmore, Madras 600 008, Tamil Nadu
Phone: +9144 825 0424
Fax: +9144 825 6336

Secretary-General
Prof. M. C. Maheshwari
Dept. of Neurology, Neurosciences Ctr.,
All India Institute of Medical Sciences
Ansari Nagar
New Delhi, 110 029
Phone: +9111 686 4851/4856
Fax: +9111 686 2663
E-mail maheshwa@medinst.ernet.in

Indonesia
Prof. Sidiarto Kusumoputro
President, Indonesian Society Against Epilepsy
c/o Bag. Neurologi F.K.U.I./R.S.C.M.

Jl. Salemba 6
Jakarta
Phone: +6221 39 17 349
Fax: +6221 31 49 424

Secretary-General
Lily D. Sidiarto, M. D.
Jl. Jelita Utara No. 11
Rawamangun
Jakarta 13220
Phone: +6221 335 044
E-mail sidiarto@indo.net.id

Ireland
Dr. John Kirker
President, Irish Chapter of the ILAE
St. Michael's Private Clinic
Crofton Road, Dun Laoghaire, Co.
Dublin
Phone: +353 1 8450243
Fax: +353 1 4557013

Secretary-General
Deirdre McMackin
Beaumont Hospital
Dublin 9

Israel
Prof. Meir Bialer
President, Israeli Chapter of the ILAE
The Hebrew University of Jerusalem
Faculty of Medicine, School of Pharmacy
P. O. Box 12065, Ein Karem
Jerusalem 91120
Phone: +972 26758610
Fax: +972 26436246 or +972 26784010
E-mail bialer@md2.huji.ac.il

Vice-President
Dr. Miri Neufeld
Dept. of Neurology
Tel-Aviv Souraski Medical Center
Tel-Aviv 64239

Italy
Prof. Claudio Munari
Presidente, Lega Italiana contro l'Epilessia
Centro Reg. per la Chirurgia dell'Epilessia

Osp. Niguarda
Piazza Ospedale Maggiore 3
I - 20126 Milan
Phone: +392 6444 2917/8
Fax: +392 6444 2868

Secretary
Prof. Federico Vigevano
Divisione di Neurofisiologia
Ospedale Bambino Gesù
Piazza S. Onofrio, 4
I - 00165 Roma
Phone: +396 685 92451
Fax: +396 685 92463
E-mail vigevano@opbg.net

Japan
Kazuichi Yagi, M. D.
President, Japan Epilepsy Society
c/o National Epilepsy Center
Shizuoka Higashi Hospital
886 Urushiyama, Shizuoka 420
Phone: +81 54 245 54 46
Fax: +81 54 246 18 80

Jordan
Prof. Ashraf Al Kurdi
President, Jordanian Chapter of Epilepsy
Jordan Medical Council
P. O. Box 5025
Amman, 11183
Phone: +9626 644544
Fax: +9626 615500

Latvia
Egils Vitols, M. D.
President, Latvian League against Epilepsy
Medical Academy of Latvia
Dept. of Neurology, Hospital No. 7 of Riga
Hipokrata Srt. 2
LV - 1038 Riga
Phone: +3717 539524
Fax: +3712 539524

Secretary:
Jana Mutazala, M. D.
Latvian League against Epilepsy

Medical Academy of Latvia
Dzirnavu St. 62-10
LV-1050 Riga

Lithuania
Prof. Egidijus Juozas Jarñemskas
President, The Society of Epileptologists of Lithuania,
Dept. of Neurosurgery, Vilnius University Emergency Hosp.
Siltnamiu 29
2043 Vilnius
Phone: +3702 26 92 48
Fax: +3702 26 89 80
E-mail egijar@kaunas.omnitel.net
        ejarzemskas@hotmail.com

Secretary
Milda Endziniene, M. D.
Neurological Clinic
Kaunas Medical Academy
Mickeviiaus 9
3000 Kaunas
Phone: +3707 79 95 72
Fax: +3707 22 07 33, +3707 79 26 27

Macedonia
Prof. Dr. M. Pashu
President
Macedonian League against Epilepsy
Dept. of Clinical Neurophysiology
Clinic of Neurology, Faculty of Medicine
Vodnjanska 17
91000 Skopje

Executive Officer
Prof. Dr. N. Sofijanov
Dept. of Child Neurology
Pediatric Clinic of the Faculty of Medicine
Vodnjanska 17
91000 Skopje
Phone: +389 91 229156
Fax:. +389 91 229156

Mexico
Dr. Juan Márquez Padilla
Presidente, Capítulo Mexicano de la ILAE
Calle Jesús García N° 2447
Colonia Ladrón de Guevara

Guadalajara Jalisco, C. P. 44640
Phone: +523 641 6233
Fax: +523 641 6233

Secretary
Dr. Agní Orozco Vázquez
Calle Día N° 2740
Jardines del Bosque
Guadalajara Jalisco, C. P. 44520

Moldova
Prof. Stanislav Groppa
President
Moldavian League against Epilepsy
Medical State University „N. Testemitsanu"
Cuza Voda str. 43 - 36
2072 Kishinau
Phone: +3732 76 37 02
Fax: +3732 2462 64
E-mail groppa@ch.moldpac.md

Secretary
V. Lisnic
Gh. Asachi str. 60/1 - 31
2028 Kishinau

Morocco
Prof. Reda Ouazzani
Président
Ligue Marocaine contre l'Épilepsie
Service de Neurophysiologie Clinique
Hôpital des Spécialités
Rabat

The Netherlands
Dr. W. O. Renier
President, Nederlandse Liga tegen Epilepsie
University Hospital of Nijmegen
Institute of Neurology - I K N C (354)
P, O, Box 9101
NL - 6500 HB Nijmegen
Phone: +31 24 361 4894
Fax: +31 24 361 7018

Office
Nederlandse Liga Tegen Epilepsie
P. O. Box 270
NL - 3990 GB Houten

Phone: +31 30 63 440 63
Fax: +31 30 63 440 60

Norway

Svein I. Johannessen, Ph. D.
President, Norwegian Chapter of the ILAE
Statens Senter for Epilepsi
P.O. Box 900
N - 1301 Sandvika
Phone: +47 67 55 41 69
Fax: +47 67 54 04 96
E-mail svein@epilepsy.no

Panamá

Dr. Ernesto Triana
President, Liga Panameña contra la Epilepsia
Apartado 6-9664
El Dorado, Panamá
Phone: +507 260 0819
Fax: +507 260 0819

Secretary
Dr. Luis Carlos Castillo
LIPACE
Apdo. 1439-9A
Carrasquilla
Fax: +507 61 55 25

Perú

Dr. Javier Florez Del Aguila
Presidente, Liga Peruana contra la Epilepsia
Avenida 2 de Mayo 649
San Isidro - Lima 27

Secretary
Dra. Patricia Campos Olazabal
Neurología, Neuropediatría
Orbi-Médica S. A.
Avda. 2 de Mayo 649
San Isidro - Lima 27
Phone: +51 14 417 950 or +511 461 5014
Fax: +51 14 822 610

Poland

Prof. Jerzy Majkowski
President, Polish League against Epilepsy
Wietnicza 122
00 - 952 Warsaw

Poland
Phone: +4822 422 492
Fax: +4822 642 7434
E-mail fund_epi_jm@zigzag.pl

Secretary
Dr. Piotr Zwoliöski
Dept. of Neurol. a. Epileptology
Med. Center for Postgr. Education
ul. Czerniakowska 231
00-416 Warszawa
Phone: +4822 629 4349
Fax: +4822 625 1014

Portugal
Dr. Francisco Pinto
President, Portuguese League against Epilepsy
Consulta de Epilepsia, Serviço de Neurologia,
Hospital Santa Maria
Avenida Prof. Egas Moniz
1600 Lisboa
Phone: +3511 797 5171
Fax: +3511 797 1321

Secretary-General
Dr. Dílio Alves
Neurology Service
Hospital Pedro Hispano
Matosinhos
4150 Porto
Fax: +3512 3322121

Romania
Ioan-Radu Rogozea, M. D., Ph. D.
President, Romanian Society against Epilepsy
Hospital "Prof. D. Bagdasar",
I Neurosurgical Clinic, Dept. of Epilepsy
Sos. Berceni No. 10, OP 8, Sect. 4
75622 Bucharest
Phone: +401 683 20 55
Fax: +401 330 72 82

Secretary
Vladimir Moldoveanu
Str. C. Georgian, Nr. 16, Sect. 2
Bucharest

Russia
Prof. George S. Burd +
President, Russian League against Epilepsy
1st City Hospital, Dept. of Neurology and
Neurosurgery
Russian State Medical University
Leninsky pr., 8, block 8
117049 Moscow

Secretary-General
Alla B. Guekht, M. D., Ph. D.
Prospect Mira 118A apt. 46
129164 Moscow
Phone: +7095 2874966
Fax: +7095 2621999 or +7095 1512651
E-mail A.Shpak@g23.relcom.ru

Kingdom of Saudi Arabia
Dr. Salch Al Deeb
President, Saudi Chapter of Epilepsy
Riyadh Armed Forces Hospital
P. O. Box 7897
Riyadh 1159
Phone: +9661 477 7714
Fax: +9661 477 7194

Secretary
Dr. Basim Yaqub
Riyadh Armed Forces Hospital
P. O. Box 7897
Riyadh 1159
Phone: +9661 477 7714
Fax: +9661 477 7194

Slovakia
Vladimir Donáth, M. D., Ph. D.
President, Slovak League against Epilepsy
Department of Neurology
F. D. Roosevelt Hospital
97517 Banská Bystrica
Phone: +421 88 41303 97 or +421 88 441 2138
Fax: +421 88 41303 97
E-mail vdonath@isternet.sk

Slovenia
Prof. Dusan Butinar
President, Slovenian League Against Epilepsy

Institute of Clinical Neurophysiology
University Medical Centre
1525 Ljubljana
Phone: +386 61 316 152 or +386 61 1313 206
Fax: +386 61 302 771
E-mail dusan.butinar@mf.uni-lj.si

Vice-President
Dr. Igor M. Ravnik
Centre for Epilepsy, Pediatriöna Klinika
Vrazov trg 1
61104 Ljubljana
Phone: +386 61 124 124
Fax: +386 61 310 246

Spain
Dr. Antonio Russi
President, Liga Española contra la Epilepsia
Centro Médico Teknon
Marquesa Vilallonga, 12 (46)
E - 08017 Barcelona
Phone: +3493 415 7577
Fax: +3493 415 7220
E-mail 6764art@comb.es

Secretariat
Dr. Santiago Arroyo
Madrazo 33 - 37, 4. 3.
E - 08006 Barcelona
Phone: +3493 415 7577
Fax: +3493 415 7220

Sweden
Kristina Malmgren, M. D., Ph. D.
President, Swedish Epilepsy Society
Neur divisionen, klinikomr 5
Sahlgrenska sjukhuset
S - 413 45 Göteborg
Phone: +46 31 342 2763
Fax: +46 31 342 2467
E-mail kristina.malmgren@neu.gu.se

Secretary
Ingrid Olsson, M. D.
Barnklinik
Östra sjukhuset
S - 416 85 Göteborg

Phone: +46 31 37 47 30
Fax: +46 31 25 79 60

Switzerland

Prof. Dr. med. P. A. Despland
Präsident, Schweizerische Liga gegen Epilepsie (SLgE)
Dorfstrasse 2, Postfach 233
CH - 8712 Stäfa/ZH
Phone: +411 926 8971
Fax: +411 926 8972

Office
Esther Hobi-Scherer
Schweizerische Liga gegen Epilepsie
Dorfstrasse 2, Postfach 233
CH - 8712 Stäfa/ZH
Phone: +411 926 8971
Fax: +411 926 8972
E-mail SlgE@bluewin.ch

Taiwan

Dr. Chun-Hing Yiu
President, Taiwan Epilepsy Society
Neurological Institute, Section of Epilepsy
The Veterans General Hospital-Taipei,
201, Shih-Pai Road, Section 2
Taipei, Taiwan 112
Phone: +8862 28757587
Fax: +8862 28762891

Secretary-General
Der-Jing Yen M. D.
Epilepsy Section, Neurological Institute
Veterans General Hospital-Taipei
201, Shih-Pai Road, Section 2
Taipei, Taiwan 112
Phone: +8862 28762890
Fax: +8862 28762891

Thailand

Prof. Pongsakdi Visudhiphan
President, Epilepsy Society of Thailand
Dept. of Pediatrics, Faculty of Medicine
Ramathibodi Hospital, Mahidol University
Rama VI Road
Bangkokg 10400
Phone: +662 2456068 or +662 2011488
Fax: +662 2011850 or +662 2462123

Tunisia
Prof. Amel Mrabet
President, Tunisian Association Against Epilepsy (TAAE)
Neurological Department
E. P. S. Charles Nicolle
Tunis 1006
Phone: +216 1 562 834
Fax: +216 1 562 777 and 562 834

Secretary General
Pr. Najoua Miladi
16, Rue 6488 Romana II
Le Bardo
Phone: +216 1 663 540
Fax: +216 1 516 579

Turkey
Dr. Esat Eökazan
President, Epilepsy Society of Turkey
Cerrahpaöa Tip Fakültesi
Farmakoloji Department
Istanbul
Phone: +90212 586 1552
Fax: +90212 633 0131

Secretary-General
Çidem Özkara, M. D.
CerrahpaÕaTip Fakültesi
Nöroloji A. B. D.
I-7-C-27 7-8. Kisim Ataköy
34750 Istanbul
Phone: +90212 633 0176
Fax: +90212 633 0176
E-mail cozkara@sim.net.tr

Ukraine
Ludmila E. Mouzichouk, M. D.
President
Ukrainian League against Epilepsy
Epilepsy Centre
Scientific Medical Centre/Psychiatry
103^A Frunze Str.
254 655 Kyiv
Phone: +380 44 435 2127
Fax: +380 44 435 3217 or +380 44 213 3431

Secretary:
Galina L. Maryek, M. D.
Epilepsy Centre
Scientific Medical Centre/Psychiatry
103^A Frunze Str.
254 655 Kyiv
Phone: +380 44 435 2127
Fax: +380 44 435 3217

Uruguay
Dr. Alejandro Scaramelli
Presidente, Liga Uruguaya contra la Epilepsia
Hospital de Clínicas, Piso 2
Av. Italia s/n
11600 Montevideo
Phone: +5982 80 12 21 and +5982 95 96 25
Fax: +5982 80 84 23
E-mail scaram@adinet.com.uy

Secretary:
Dra. Isabel Rega
Liga Uruguaya contra la Epilepsia LUCE
Instituto de Neurología
Hospital de Clínicas, Piso 2
Av Italia s/n
1160 Montevideo

USA
Robert L. Macdonald, M. D., Ph. D.
President, American Epilepsy Society
Univers. of Michigan; Neuroscience Lab. Building
1103 East Huron Street
Ann Arbor, MI 48104-1687
Phone: +1 313 763 3720
Fax: +1 313 763 7686

Office
American Epilepsy Society
638 Prospect Avenue
Hartford, CT 06105-4298
Phone: +1 860 586 7505
Fax: +1 860 586 7550
E-mail info@aesnet.org

Venezuela
Dra. Beatriz González del Castillo
Presidenta, Liga Venezolana Contra la Epilepsia

Quebrada Honda a Santa Rosa
Edificio Táchira, Planta Baja, Mariperg
Caracas 1040
Phone: +582 5763081 or +582 5762619
        +582 5728370
E-mail beacastle@telcel.net.ve

Secretary
Dra. Euse Beatriz Blanco Montes
Liga Venezolana contra la Epilepsia
Quebrada Honda a Santa Rosa
Edificio Táchira, Planta Baja, Mariperg
Caracas 1040
Phone: +582 5763081 or +582 5762619
        +582 5728370

Yugoslavia
Dr. Dragoslav V. Ercegovac
President
Yugoslav Union of Leagues against Epilepsy
Center for Epileptology and Migraine
Brae Jugovia Str. 14/I
11000 Beograd
Phone: +381 11 63 10 54
Fax: +381 11 63 10 54
E-mail ercegovd@EUnet.yu

Provisionally accepted chapters:

Armenia
Prof. Vahagn Darbinyan, M. D.
President, Armenian National League against Epilepsy
Institute of Surgery
9, Asratyan St., Kanaker
375052 Yerevan
Phone: +3742 284401
E-mail: vdarb@ipia.sci.am

Secretary-General:
Kteyan Armina A., M. D.
Armenian Republican Epilepsy Center
State Medical University
Institute of Surgery
9, Asratyan St.,
375052 Yerevan

Phone: +3742 284652
E-mail: epilepsy@acc.am

Estonia
Sulev Haldre
President, Estonian League Against Epilepsy
Dept. of Neurology and Neurosurgery
University of Tartu
2 Puusepp Str.
EE-2400 Tartu
Phone: +3727 448500/02
Fax: +3727 448509
E-mail: sulev@cut.ee

Secretary
Andre Öun
Dept. of Neurology and Neurosurgery
University of Tartu
2 Puusepp Str.
EE-2400 Tartu
Phone: +3727 448545
Fax: +3726 448509
E-mail: andre@cut.ee

Malta
Anthony Galea Debono, M. D.
President, Epilepsy Society of Malta
St. Luke's Hospital
G'Mangia
Phone: +356 2595 1411
Fax: +356 3732 37

Secretary
Janet Mifsud, B. Pharm, Ph. D.
Dept. of Clinical Pharmacology and Therapeutics
University of Malta
Msida, MSD 06
Phone: +356 32902910 and +356 32902845
Fax: +356 320281
E-mail: janmif@cis.um.edu.mt

Senegal
Prof. I. Pierre Ndiaye
President, Ligue Senegalaise contre l'Epilepsie
Clinique Neurologique
CHU Fann
B. P. 5035

Dakar
Phone: +221 251930
Fax: +221 252952

1st Vice-President
Prof. Mamadou Gueye
Clinique Neurologique
CHU Fann
B. P. 5035
Dakar
Phone: +221 251930
Fax: +221 252952

Syria
Dr. Ahmad Khalifa
President, Syrian Chapter of Epilepsy
P. O. Box 10053
Damascus
Phone: +96311 3310600
Fax: +96311 3322922

International Bureau for Epilepsy
Office
P.O. Box 21
NL – 2100 AA Heemstede
The Netherlands
Fax: +3123 547 0119
Email: ibe@xs411.nl

President:
Richard Holmes
253 Crumlin Road
Dublin 12, Ireland
Fax: +353 1455 4648
Email: tiec@indigo.ie

Chapters

Argentina
Associacion de Lucha contra la Epilepsia
Tucuman 3261
CP 1189 Buenos Aires
Tel: +54 1 8620 440
Fax: +54 1 8634 350

Australia
National Epilepsy Association of Australia

Suite 2B 44-46 Oxford Street
PO Box 879
Epping
NSW 2121
Tel: +61 298 698 444
Fax: +61 298 694 122
Email: epilepsy @nectar.com.au

Austria
Epilepsie Selbsthilfegruppen Osterreichs
Haupstr. 44/2/2
2344 Ma Enzersdorf

Belgium
Belgische Nationale Bond tegen Epilepsie
Avenue Albert 135
Brussels 1060
Tel: +322 344 3263
Fax: +322 346 1193

Canada
Epilepsy Canada
1470 Peel Street, Suite 745
Montreal
Quebec H3A ITI
Tel: +1 514 845 7855
Fax: +1 514 845 7866
Email: epilepsy@epilepsy.ca

Chile
Liga contra la Epilepsia de Valparaiso
Alvares 1532
Casilla 705 (Hospital G. Fricke)
Vina del Mar

Colombia
Liga Colombiana contra la Epilepsia
Cap de Bolivar
Barrio Ternera
calle la El Eden
Y 5007 Cartagena
Tel: +57 566 18 107
Fax: +57 566 18 111
Email: fandino@cartagena.cetcol.net.co

Croatia
Croatian Association for Epilepsy
Department of Paediatrics

Division of Neuropediatrics
University Hospital Center Rebro
Kispaticevia 12
10 000 Zagreb
Tel: +385 121 3087
Fax: +385 121 0900

Cuba
Cuban Chapter IBE
Sociedad de Neurociencias de Cuba
Seccion de Epilepsia
Hospital Psiquiatrico de la Habana
Ave Independencia No 26520
Rpio Mazorra Ap 9
Boyoros, Cuidad de la Habana
CP 19220
Tel: +537 451 688
Fax: +537 451 512

Czech Republic
Czech Epilepsy Association
Spolecnost "E"
Novodvorska 994
CZ 14221 Prague
Tel/Fax: +4202 4404 1557
Fax: +4202 4723 464

Denmark
Dansk Epilepsiforening
Dr Sellsvej 28
DK 4293 Dianalund
Tel: +45 5826 44 66
Fax: +45 5826 44 51

Ecuador
Asociacion de Padres de Ninos con Epilepsia
Isla Marchena 300 y Los Granados
PO Box 17-15-221 C
Quito
Fax: +00 593 246 9141
Email: gbpesantez@puceuio.puce.edu.ec

Finland
Epilepsyaliitto
Malmin Kauppatie 26
FIN-00700 Helsinki
Tel: +358 9350 82320

Fax: +358 9350 82322

France
AISPACE
11 Avenue Kennedy
F-59800 Lille
Tel No: +33 320 571 941
Fax No: +33 2009 4124

Germany
Deutsche Epilepsie Vereinigung
ZillestraBe 102
10585 Berlin
Tel: +49 30 342 4414
Fax: +49 30 342 4466

Ghana
Ghana Epilepsy Association
c/o PO Box M230
Accra

Greece
Greek National Association against Epilepsy
Aghia Sophia Children's Hospital
Dept. of Neurology/Neurophysiology
Athens 11527
Tel: +30 177 718 11
Fax: +30 177 057 85

Hungary
Hungarian Epilepsy Association (HALE)
1028 Budapest
Hidegkuti ut 71
Tel/Fax: +36 1 393 28829

Iceland
The Epilepsy Association of Iceland
Postbox 5182
126 Reykjavik
Tel: +354 551 4570
Fax: +354 813 552

India
Indian Epilepsy Association
8 Palam Marg,
Vasant Vihar
New Delhi 110057
Tel: +91 124 35 00 35

Indonesia
PERPEI
Jl. Jelita Utara No.11
Rawamangun
Jakarta 13220
Fax: +62 21 797 0533

Iran
Iranian Epilepsy Association
PO Box 15655/199
Tehran
Fax: +98 75 33 847

Ireland
Brainwave The Irish Epilepsy Association
249 Crumlin Road
Dublin 12
Tel: +353 1 455 75 00
Fax: +353 1 455 70 13
Email: brainwve@iol.ie

Israel
EYAL
Israel Epilepsy Association
4 Avodat Yisrael St, PO Box 1598
Jerusalem 91014
Tel: +972 2537 1044
Fax: +972 2653 5508

Italy
Associazione Italiana contro l'Epilessia (AICE)
Via T. Marino No 7
20121 Milano
Tel: +39 2 809 299
Fax: +39 2 809 799

Japan
The Japan Epilepsy Association
5F Zenkokuzaidan Building 2-2-8
Nishiwaseda
Shinjuku-ku
Tokyo 162
Tel: +81 332 025 661
Fax: +81 332 027 235

Kenya
Kenya Association for the Welfare of Epileptics
PO Box 60790

Nairobi
Tel: +254 257 0885

Korea
Korean Epilepsy Association/Rose Club
157-1 Saejong-ro
Jongro-ku
Seoul 110-021
Tel: +822 394 2375
Fax: +822 394 7169

Malaysia
Persatuan Epilepsi Malaysia
Jabatan Neurologi
Hospital Besar
50586 Kuala Lumpur
Fax: +60 329 48 187

Mexico
Groupo "Aceptacion" de Epilepticos
Amsterdam 1928 No 19
Colonia Olimpica-Pedregal
Mexico 04710 DF
Fax: +525 575 3250

The Netherlands
Epilepsie Vereniging Nederland
PO Box 270
3990 GB Houten
Tel: +31 306 344 063
Fax: +31 306 344 060

New Zealand
Epilepsy Association of New Zealand Inc
PO Box 1074
Hamilton
Tel: +64 7834 3556
Fax: +64 7834 3553

Norway
Norsk Epilepsiforbund
Storgt. 39
0182 Oslo
Tel: +47 2220 6021
Fax: +47 2211 5976

Peru
Peruvian Association of Epilepsy

Castilla 678-E 101
Lima 32
Fax: +51 1 466 0063
Email: capnlp@mail01.protelsa.com.pe

Poland
Polskie Stowarzyszenie
Ludzi Cierpiacych na Padaczke
15-482 Bialystok
Ul.Fabryczna 57 (Xlp.)
Tel/Fax: +48 85754 420

Portugal
Liga Portuguesa contra a Epilepsia
Rua Sa da Bandeira 162-1 o
4000 Porto
Fax: +351 233 22 121

Senegal
Ligue Senegalaise contre l'Epilepsie
Clinique Neurologique
Centre Hospitalo-Universitaire de Fann
BP 5035
Dakar-Fann

Scotland
Epilepsy Association of Scotland
48 Govan Road
Glasgow G51 1JL
Tel: +44 141 427 4911
Fax: 44 141 419 1709

Singapore
Singapore Epilepsy Foundation
2 Finlayson Green #16/05
Asian Insurance Building
Singapore 049247
Tel: +65 222 8291
Fax: +65 222 3041

Slovenia
Liga Proti Epilepsiji Slovenije
Institute of Clinical Neurophysiology
Hospital of Neurology
Medical Centre
SI-1525 Ljubljana
Tel: +38 661 131 3206
Fax: +38 661 302 771

South Africa
South African National Epilepsy League
SANEL PO Box 73
Observatory 7935
Tel: +27 214 730 014
Fax: +27 214 485 053

Spain
PENEPA
Calle Excuelas Pias n.89
Barcelona 08017
Tel: +34 334 954 00
Fax: +34 341 849 22

Sri Lanka
Epilepsy Association of Sri Lanka
10 Austin Place
Colombo 8
Tel: +94 1696 283

Sweden
Svenska Epilepsiforbundet
PO Box 9514
102 74 Stockholm
Tel: +46 866 943 06
Fax: +46 866 915 88
Email: susanne.lund@epilepsi.se

Switzerland
Dorfstrasse 2
Postfach 233
8712 Stafa/ZH
Zurich
Switzerland

Taiwan
Taiwan Epilepsy Association
c/o Division of Epilepsy
Dept. of Neurology
Chang Gung Memorial Hospital
199 Tun-Hwa N. Road
Taipei 105
Tel: +88 633 28 1200 ext.2249
Fax: +88 633 28 1320

Tunisia
Tunisian Association Against Epilepsy
Neurological Dept.

EPS Charles Nicolle
Tunis 1006
Tel: +216 1 562 834
Fax: +216 1 562 777

UK
British Epilepsy Association
Anstey House
40 Hanover Square
Leeds LS3 IBE
Tel: +44 113 243 9393
Fax: +44 113 242 8804
Email: epilepsy@bea.org.uk

USA
Epilepsy Foundation
4351 Garden City Drive
Landover, Maryland 20785
Tel: +1 301 459 3700
Fax: +1 301 577 2684
Email: postmaster @efa.org

Yugoslavia
Jugoslovensko Drustvo za Epilepsiju
Yugoslav Society for Epilepsy
Slobodana Penezica-Krcuna 23
Beograd
Belgrade
Tel: +381 11 68 61 55 ext. 137
Fax: +381 11 68 66 56
Email: yusepi@rhc.ztp.co.yu

Zimbabwe
Epilepsy Support Foundation
PO Box A104 Avondale
Old General Hospital
Mazoe Street
Harare
Tel: +263 472 4071

Friends

Brazil
Brazilian Association of Epilepsy
UNICAMP – Cx Postal: 6138
CEP: 13.081-970 Campinas SP

Tel: +55 192 39 7990
Fax: +55 192 52 6773

Brazil
Associacione Catarinense de Epilepsia
Rua Esteves Junior
390-1 o andar Bloco M
Florianopolis SC 88015-530

Cameroon
Epilepsy Research and Action Center
BP 14606
Yaounde
Tel: +237 31 6505
Fax: +237 31 6505
Email: ERAC@Cam.Healthnet.Org

Denmark
Dianalund Epilepsy Hospital
DK 4293 Dianalund
Tel: +45 356 4200

Ecuador
Liga Tunguruense de Control de la Epilepsia
Mera 5-27 y Sucre, Segundo Piso
Ambato

France
Bureau Francais de l'Epilepsie
236 bis, rue de Tolbiac
75013 Paris
Tel: +33 1 53 60 6664
Fax: +33 1 45 30 0809

Indonesia
Yayasan Epilepsi Indonesia
Indonesian Epilepsy Foundation
Jl Senayan No 16 Blok S
Kebayoran Baru
Jakarta Selatan 12180
Tel/Fax: +62 21 722 0621

Israel
Association of Epileptics in Israel
PO Box 5355
Herzlia 46101
Tel: +972 9508 152
Fax: +972 9580 627

Japan
National Epilepsy Centre
Shizuoka Higashi Hospital
886 Urushiyama
Shizuoka 420
Tel: +81 542 455 446
Fax: +81 542 461 880

Japan
Epilepsy Hospital Bethel
27-4 Hata-Mukaiyama-Minami
Kitahase
Iwanuma City 989-24
Tel: +81 223 241 211
Fax: +81 223 242 265

Korea
Songpo Epilepsy Foundation
#302 Dongil B/D
Insadong, Chongro-Ku
Seoul, 110-290
Tel: +822 735 777 35
Fax: +882 732 8717

The Netherlands
Dr Hans Berger Kliniek
Galderseweg 81
Postbus 90108
4800 RA Breda
Tel: +31 76 5608 200
Fax: +31 76 5608 287

The Netherlands
Nationaal Epilepsie Fonds/De Macht van het Kleine
Postbus 270
3990 GB Houten
Tel: +31 30 63 440 63
Fax: +31 30 63 440 60

The Netherlands
Instituut voor Epilepsiebestrijding
Meer and Bosch/De Cruquiushoeve
PO Box 21
2100 AA Heemstede
Tel: +31 23 523 7237
Fax: +31 23 529 4324

The Netherlands
Stichting Kempenhaeghe
Sterkselseweg 65
5591 VE Heeze
Tel: +31 4907 790 22
Fax: +31 4907 649 24

Scotland
Enlighten
5 Coates Place
Edinburgh
EH3 7AA
Tel: +44 131 226 5458
Fax: +44 131 220 2855
Email: enlighten@cableinet.co.uk

Switzerland
Par Epi
Waldhofstrasse 21
CH 6314 Unterageri
Tel: +41 41 750 5002
Fax: + 41 41 750 4034

Switzerland
Swiss Epilepsy Centre
Bleulerstrasse 60
CH-8008 Zurich
Tel: +41 1387 61 11
Fax: +41 1387 62 49

UK
Epilepsi Cymru-Epilepsy Wales
15 Chester Street
St. Asaph
Denbighshire LL17 ORE
Tel/Fax: +44 174 558 4444

UK
David Lewis Centre for Epilepsy
Near Alderley Edge
Cheshire SK9 7UD
Tel: +44 1565 872 613
Fax: +44 1565 872 829

UK
The National Society for Epilepsy
Chalfont Centre for Epilepsy

Chalfont St. Peter
Gerrards Cross
Bucks SL9 ORJ
Tel: +44 149 487 3991
Fax: +44 149 487 1927

UK
Gravesend Epilepsy Network
13 St. George's Cresent
Gravesend
Kent DA12 4AR
Tel: +44 147 435 1673
Fax: +44 147 485 5946

UK
St. Piers Lingfield
St. Piers Lane
Lingfield
Surrey RH7 6PW
Tel: +44 1342 832 243
Fax: +44 1342 834 639

Other
World Health Organization
1211 Geneva 27 Switzerland
Tel: 00 41 22 791 2111
Fax: 00 41 22 791 0746

Resource AD

Literature for the Waiting Room

1. *Epigraph*, an international epilepsy newsletter, The National Society for Epilepsy, Chalfont St Peter, Bucks, SL9 ORJ, UK

2. Epilepsy Foundation Catalog, Books, Videos, Guides and Pamphlets, National Office, 4351 Garden City Drive, Landover, MD 20785-2267

3. Epilepsy Foundation Poster, Medicines for Epilepsy, a wall chart with color photographs of antiepileptic medications

4. Keto Klub Quarterly Newsletter, Keto Klub, Inc., A Non-Profit Corporation, 61557 Miami Meadows Court, South Bend, IN, 46614

Resource AE

Summer Camps for Children with Epilepsy

Alabama
Camp Candlelight at Camp ASCCA
Epilepsy Foundation of North and Central Alabama and Epilepsy
Chapter of Mobile and Gulf Coast
Ages 6–16
Michele Robertson
(800) 950-6662
(205) 870-1146
Charlotte Van Erman
(800) 626-1582
(334) 432-0970

Arizona
Camp Candlelight at Shadow Pines
Epilepsy Foundation of Arizona
Ages 8–15
Dean Crafton
(888) 768-2670
(602) 406-3581

California
Camp Quest
Epilepsy Society of San Diego County
Optimist Clubs, and MECRO
Ages 8–14
Jackie Vella
(619) 296-0161

Connecticut
Camp Hemlocks
Epilepsy Foundation of Connecticut
Ages 8–12
Bonnie McAneny
(800) 899-3745
(860) 721-9226

Florida
Boggy Creek Gang Camp
Epilepsy Foundation of NE Florida, Epilepsy Foundation of Eastern
Florida, Epilepsy Foundation of South Florida, and Epilepsy Founda-
tion of SW Florida
Ages 7–15
Patricia Dean, RN, MSN
(305) 663-6819

Georgia
Camp Toccoa and Others
Georgia Chapter, EFA and Atlanta Rotary
Ages 7–18
Johnie Hall
(800) 527-7105
(404) 527-7155

Illinois
Camp Blackhawk
Epilepsy Foundation of Greater Chicago and Epilepsy Association of
Rock Valley
Ages 8–16
Mary Kolovitz
(800) 273-6027
(312) 939-8622
Cara Witkowski
(800) 221-2689
(815) 964-2689/extension 22

Camp ROEHR
Epilepsy Foundation of Southwestern Illinois, Ortho-McNeil, Comprehensive Epilepsy Care of St. Luke's Hospital
Ages 7–12
Michelle Kilian
Peggy Mueller
(618) 236-2181

Maryland
Chesapeake Center
Epilepsy Foundation of the Chesapeake Region and the Chesapeake
Center
Ages 7–15
Sabrina Cooke
(410) 828-7700
(800) 492-2523

Michigan
Camp Discovery
Epilepsy Foundation of Michigan
YMCA Camp Storer
Ages 3–7
The Fowler Center
Ages 8–18
Reginna Chidester
(248) 351-2102/extension 231
(800) 377-6226

Minnesota
Camp Oz
Epilepsy Foundation of Minnesota, Gillette Children's Specialty
Healthcare and Epilepsy Clinical Research Program at the University of
Minnesota
Ages 8–17
Deb McNally
(612) 646-8675
(800) 779-0777

Mississippi
Alvin P. Flannes Camp
Epilepsy Foundation of Mississippi
Ages 9–13
Beth McLarty
(601) 362-2761
(800) 898-0291

Missouri
Camp Shing
Epilepsy Foundation Heart of America
Ages 6–16
Susan Stanton
(816) 444-2800
(800) 972-5163

New Jersey
Camp NOVA
Epilepsy Foundation of New Jersey
Ages 8–25
Renee Davidson
(609) 858-5900

New York
Camp EAGR
Epilepsy Foundation of Rochester and Syracuse Regions
Ages 8–15
Joan P. Powell
(800) 724-7930
(716) 442-4430

Ohio
Camp Dream Catcher
Epilepsy Council of Greater Cincinnati
Ages 7–17
Mark Findley
(513) 721-2905

Achievement Center for Children—Camp Cheerful
Epilepsy Foundation of Northeast Ohio
Ages 7–12
Alice Weil
(216) 579-1330

Pennsylvania
Camp Frog
Epilepsy Foundation of Western Pennsylvania
Ages 9–18
Beth Lott
(800) 361-5885
(412) 261-5880

Puerto Rico
Encuentro Recreativo y Educacional de Epilepsia
Sociedad Puertorriqueña de Ayuda al Paciente con Epilepsia, Parke-
Davis, Glaxo Wellcome, and Fondos Unidos de Puerto Rico
Ages 5–16 and 17–27 (necesidades especiales)
Nydia I. Echevarria
Gloria M. Ramos
Yimar Santos
(787) 782-6200

South Carolina
Camp River Run
Epilepsy Foundation of South Carolina
Ages 7–14
Christine Porter
(803) 929-3948
(803) 733-6210

Tennessee
Camp Lakewood
Epilepsy Foundation of Greater Chattanooga and Kiwanis Club of Chat-
tanooga
Ages 7–16
Theresa Ingram
(423) 756-1771

Texas
Camp Spike-n-Wave
Ages 8–14
Kamp Kaleidoscope
Ages 15–19
Epilepsy Foundation of Southeast Texas
Heather Boyd or Tracy Hurst
(713) 789-6295

Camp Summit
Ages 7–17
Epilepsy Foundation of Greater North Texas
Ginny Schwindt
(214) 823-8809

Washington
Camp Discovery
Epilepsy Association of Washington
Ages 6–16
Yolanda Larson
(206) 547-4551
(800) 752-3509

Wisconsin
Camp Phoenix
Epilepsy Center South Central
Ages 8–15
Jane Boltz
Art Taggart
(608) 833-8888
(800) 657-4929

Glossary of Acronyms

Glossary of Acronyms

ACTH:	adrenocorticotropic hormone
ADA:	Americans with Disabilities Act
AED:	antiepileptic drug
AMPA:	a-amino-3-hydroxy-5-methylisoxazole-4-propionic acid
BEOP:	benign epilepsy with occipital paroxysms
BECRS:	benign epilepsy of childhood with rolandic spikes
BETS:	benign epileptiform transients of sleep
BREC:	benign rolandic epilepsy of childhood (same as BECRS)
CAT:	computed axial tomography
CBZ:	carbamazepine
CCTV/EEG:	closed circuit television and electroencephalography
CNS:	central nervous system
CSWDS:	continuous spike-wave discharges during sleep
DSM-IV:	*Diagnostic and Statistical Manual of Mental Disorders,* 4th edition
DVS:	divalproex sodium (Depakote)
EEG:	electroencephalogram
EFA:	Epilepsy Foundation of America
EPC:	epilepsia partialis continua

FBM: felbamate (Felbatol)

FDG: F-fluorodeoxyglucose

FLAIR: fluid-attenuated inversion recovery

fMRI: functional magnetic resonance imaging

FIRDA: frontal intermittent rhythmic delta activity

FSH: follicle-stimulating hormone

GABA: gamma-aminobutyric acid

GTC: generalized tonic-clonic seizure (convulsion)

GnRH: gonadotrophin-releasing hormone

HH: hypothalamic hypogonadism

HHE: hemiconvulsion-hemiplegia-epilepsy syndrome

5-HIAA: 5-hydroxyindoleacetic acid

HMPAO: Tc-hexamethyl-propyleneamine-oxime

Hz: Hertz (cycles per second)

IDD: interictal dysphoric disorder

IAP: intracarotid Amytal procedure

JME: juvenile myoclonic epilepsy (of Janz), also called impul-
            sive petit mal

ILAE: International League Against Epilepsy

KSS: Kearns-Sayre syndrome

LEV: levetiracetam (Keppra)

LGS: Lennox-Gastaut syndrome

LH: luteinizing hormone

LTG: lamotrigine (Lamictal)

MEG: magnetoelectroencephalography

MELAS: mitochondrial encephalomyopathy, lactic acidosis, and
            strokelike episodes

MERRF: myoclonic epilepsy with ragged red fibers

MES: maximal electroshock

MMPI: Minnesota multiphasic personality inventory

MRI: magnetic resonance imaging

MRS: magnetic resonance spectroscopy

MTS: mesial temporal sclerosis

NAA:	N-acetyl aspartate
NCSE:	nonconvulsive status epilepticus
NES:	nonepileptic seizures
OXC:	oxcarbazepine (Trileptal)
PB:	phenobarbital
PCOS:	polycystic ovary syndrome
PET:	positron emission tomography
PHT:	phenytoin (Dilantin)
PRM:	primidone (Mysoline)
PTZ:	pentylenetetrazol
QOLIE:	quality of life in epilepsy inventory
SE:	status epilepticus
SJS:	Stevens-Johnson syndrome
SREDA:	subclinical rhythmic electrographic discharge of adults
SPECT:	single photon emission computed tomography
SSPE:	subacute sclerosing panencephalitis
SSRI:	serotonin reuptake inhibitor
SSS:	small sharp spikes
SUDEP:	sudden unexplained death in epilepsy
TAPS:	Training Applicants for Placement Success; Epilepsy Foundation's training and placement service
TCA:	tricyclic antidepressant
TGB:	tiagabine (Gabitril)
TEN:	toxic epidermal necrolysis
TLE:	temporal lobe epilepsy
TPM:	topiramate (Topamax)
TS:	tuberous sclerosis
Vd:	volume of distribution
VNS:	vagal nerve stimulator
VGB:	vigabatrin
VMA:	vanillylmandelic acid
VPA:	valproic acid (Depakene)
WADA:	intracarotid amobarbital test

Glossary of Terms

Absence Seizure: Commonly seen in children between four years old and adolescence. There is no warning or postictal period. Patients have abrupt alteration of consciousness, with staring and a blank facial expression, usually lasting less than 15 seconds. Automatisms may occur. The electroencephalogram reveals generalized 3 Hertz spike and wave.

Absence Status Epilepticus (Spike Wave Stupor): Rather than blink or stare as in an absence seizure, patients are confused. Absence status typically is seen in children, but may present in old age in patients who have never had seizures. There is a good response to intravenous diazepam.

Agyria (Lissencephaly): A type of cortical dysplasia with inadequate cortical sulcation and gyration. The cortex is smooth and thin, with most of the cortical neurons misplaced in a subcortical layer.

Aicardi Syndrome: This syndrome of mental retardation, infantile spasms, agenesis of the corpus callosum, and chorioretinal lacunae affects only females and has a high rate of early mortality. Vertebral body abnormalities are common. An intrauterine insult during gestation may be responsible.

Artifact: Electroencephalogram (EEG) signals not related to brain waves. Muscle activity, sweat, patient movement, and poor electrode contacts are common sources of artifacts. Cardiac pacemakers, intravenous infusion pumps, and telephones also can create abnormal EEG signals. Artifacts can obscure important brain signals or may be mistaken for epileptic activity. Extensive training in EEG interpretation is essential to appropriately recognize artifacts.

Astatic seizure: A drop attack that may be due to a tonic, atonic, myoclonic, or partial onset seizure. Astatic seizures most often are seen in Lennox-Gastaut syndrome and may result in injury.

Atonic Seizure: A seizure due to loss of muscle tone. The head may drop, or if postural tone is lost, the patient may fall to the ground in a "drop attack." Injury may occur, particularly to the face.

Atypical Absence Seizure: Lasts longer than a typical absence seizure, more often has tone changes, associated with an abnormal interictal electroencephalogram (EEG) and seen in patients with mental retardation. The ictal EEG is faster or slower than the 3 Hertz spike and wave seen in a typical absence seizure.

Aura: The characteristic warning that heralds a partial seizure. Actually, the aura represents focal epileptic activity and is the beginning of a seizure. Clinical symptomatology depends on the location of the epileptic discharge. For example, a mesial temporal lobe focus can elicit an aura of fear, an occipital lobe focus can cause flashing lights or spots, and a frontal lobe focus can result in contralateral motor movements.

Automatisms: Involuntary abnormal movements that occur during or after an epileptic seizure while consciousness is impaired. Patients may chew, smack their lips, swallow, rub their hands, or perform more complex movements such as walking or undressing. An automatism may be new motor activity or a continuation of preictal behavior.

Benign Epileptiform Transients of Sleep: These small spikes can be unilateral or bilateral. Also known as small sharp spikes of sleep (SSS), these benign discharges should not be confused with epileptic spikes.

Benign Familial Neonatal Convulsions: Occur primarily on days 2 and 3 after birth, these clonic and apneic seizures are dominantly inherited. Only approximately 14 percent of these infants develop epilepsy.

Benign Neonatal Convulsions: These clonic or apneic seizures occur without known cause on day 5 after birth ("fifth day fits"). The electroencephalogram may show alternating theta waves. Development is normal and seizures do not recur.

Benign Myoclonic Epilepsy in Infancy: In this rare disorder, myoclonic seizures occur in normal children in the first or second year of life. Approximately one third have a family history of seizures. Developmental delay often occurs. Seizures respond well to medication. Convulsions may occur during adolescence.

Benign Rolandic Epilepsy: Also known as benign epilepsy with centrotemporal spikes, the name refers to the large epileptic spikes seen on the electroencephalogram (EEG). Seizures begin between age 2 and 13 years and are characterized by speech arrest, salivation, and facial jerking. Hemiconvulsions and convulsions also may occur. Three quarters of the seizures occur during sleep. Neuroimaging and the neurologic examination between seizures are normal. The EEG may be positive only during sleep. Patients respond well to antiepileptic drugs, and some do not require medication. Benign rolandic epilepsy is age-related, and seizures disappear by age 16.

Burst Suppression: This electroencephalographic pattern of bursts of high voltage slow waves mixed with sharp waves or spikes followed by periods of relative flatness is most commonly seen in the comatose patient and is associated with a poor prognosis.

Catamenial Epilepsy: Some women have seizures only at the time of menstruation. Many other women note an increase in seizures in the perimenstrual (days −3 to 3), ovulatory (days 10 to 13), or latter half of their menstrual cycle. Studies report a range of 10 percent to 78 percent of women with catamenial epilepsy, depending on the magnitude of seizure increase required by the authors. These patterns become evident when women carefully document seizure frequency and menstruation on a calendar. An increase in the estradiol:progesterone ratio may be responsible for the observed increase in seizures. Identifying a hormonal link to seizure frequency may allow for more targeted treatment.

Childhood Absence Epilepsy (Petit mal, True petit mal, Pyknolepsy): Characterized by multiple staring spells, this seizure type occurs in preschool or school-aged children who otherwise are neurologically normal. Seizures may be provoked by hyperventilation. The electroencephalogram reveals generalized 3 Hertz spike and wave. Forty percent of patients also have generalized tonic-clonic seizures. Ethosuximide or valproate readily control staring spells. Children usually outgrow this syndrome, which is a type of primary generalized epilepsy (see Absence Seizure).

Clonic Seizure: Repetitive jerking of muscles during a seizure.

Comprehensive Epilepsy Program: Often found at a medical school (see Resource Q for list of United States centers), these programs combine the skills of an epileptologist, neurosurgeon, neuropsychiatrist, neuropsychologist, neuroradiologist, social worker, nurse clinician, and others in a dedicated team designed to help patients with epilepsy. A comprehensive epilepsy center can provide advanced neurodiagnostic studies such as magnetic resonance imaging (MRI), single photon emission computed tomography (SPECT), positron emission tomography (PET), and video-EEG monitoring. Investigational AEDs and other research protocols will also be available. Patients likely to benefit from a comprehensive epilepsy program are those with anatomic lesions referred for epilepsy surgery, persistent seizures despite treatment with multiple AEDs, or suspected nonepileptic seizures.

Computerized Axial Tomography: A CAT or CT scan. Multiple x-ray images taken in different planes by a movable gantry are reconstructed to provide cross-sectional views of the skull and brain. CAT scans are particularly useful when searching for calcium, blood, or skull defects.

Convulsion: A generalized tonic-clonic seizure. A partial seizure may spread to become a convulsion, or a convulsion may begin globally without a focal onset.

Corpus Callosotomy: A type of epilepsy surgery particularly used for patients who have "drop attacks" due to atonic seizures and are at risk for injury. Many of these patients have Lennox-Gastaut syndrome. When the corpus callosum is severed, epileptic discharges can no longer spread as easily from one hemisphere to the other. This surgery can greatly reduce drop attacks, but it does not improve partial seizures.

Cortical Dysplasia: Broad category of neuronal migration disorders. Examples include microdysgenesis, agyria, pachygyria, polymicrogyria, and laminar heterotopia. These developmental abnormalities often lead to childhood epilepsy.

Cytochrome P450: A hepatic enzyme system consisting of more than a dozen isoenzymes responsible for the metabolism of most AEDs. For example, cytochrome P450 3A4 metabolizes carbamazepine, while phenytoin is metabolized by cytochrome P450 2C8/9/10. Cytochrome P450 activity may be induced or inhibited by AEDs and many other drugs, affecting the rate of AED metabolism and resultant serum AED levels. The potential effect on the cytochrome P450 system should be assessed whenever a new drug is added to a patient's regimen.

Déjà Vu: A sensation that a new experience has occurred before. Déjà vu is a disturbance of higher cerebral function characteristically due to a partial seizure localized in the temporal lobe. A déjà vu sensation may occur as an aura prior to a complex partial or generalized seizure.

Depth Electrodes: Invasive electrodes used to determine the seizure focus when scalp electroencephalograms remain inconclusive. Typically, four to six electrodes are placed stereotactically into the brain under computed axial tomography or magnetic resonance imaging guidance through small holes drilled into the skull. These electrodes are associated with a small risk of hemorrhage and infection.

DigiTrace: An ambulatory electroencephalogram (EEG) monitoring system that uses digital technology. The patient has EEG electrodes connected to the scalp and then takes the DigiTrace computer home for one to several days. The device contains computer software that records background samples, spikes, electrographic seizures, and push-button events. These are later downloaded and reviewed on paper. DigiTrace can also be used with video.

Early Myoclonic Encephalopathy: Myoclonus, partial seizures, or tonic spasms begin before 3 months of age. Early myoclonic encephalopathy occurs frequently in families. The electroencephalogram reveals suppression-burst activity. This severe seizure disorder may result in death before the age of 1 year.

Electroencephalogram: first discovered by Hans Berger in 1929, the electroencephalogram (EEG) remains an essential component of all clinical neurophysiology laboratories. Human brain waves reveal levels of mental alertness, sleep stages, and the presence or absence of epileptic activity. Scalp electrodes distributed in an array over the head detect endogenous cerebral electricity, which is then filtered, amplified, and continuously recorded on paper by voltage sensitive pens. Typically, 16 channels of electrical activity from different brain areas are displayed. A standard EEG represents 20 minutes of continuous recording. Modern digital EEG machines can display brain waves on a computer screen or laser printout. Prolonged recordings can save hours or days of collected information to a computer hard drive. To enhance review, software can search the record for spikes and subclinical seizures.

Electrographic Seizures (Subclinical Seizures): Seizures detected on the electroencephalogram that do not produce clinical symptoms.

Epilepsia Partialis Continua: Focal motor seizures, usually of the face or arms, consisting of clonic movements which continue for hours or days. Consciousness is preserved. Postictal weakness occurs. Rasmussen's encephalitis is commonly responsible, but these enduring seizures may also be caused by Alper's disease, subacute type of delayed measles encephalitis, and mitochondrial encephalomyopathy with lactic acidosis and strokelike episodes.

Epilepsy with Continuous Spikes and Waves During Slow Sleep: Spike wave activity occurs during at least 85 percent of slow wave sleep. Convulsions, absences, and myoclonic seizures can occur. Behavior and speech deteriorate. Seizures disappear by puberty but mental sequelae may remain.

Epilepsy with Grand Mal Seizures on Awakening: Average age of onset is 17 years. Nearly all convulsions occur after awakening from sleep, whether in the morning or after a nap. Absence or myoclonic seizures may also be seen. This appears to be an idiopathic generalized epilepsy with genetic predisposition. Seizures respond well to antiepileptic medication but often recur when drugs are stopped.

Epilepsy with Myoclonic Absences: Absence seizures begin at a mean age of 7 years accompanied by severe clonic jerks, often with a tonic contraction. Seizures are frequent and do not respond well to therapy. Mental deterioration may occur.

Epilepsy with Myoclonic-Astatic Seizures: Absence with clonic and tonic components, astatic, myoclonic, myoclonic-astatic, and tonic-clonic seizures can occur in this childhood syndrome. Status epilepticus is frequent.

Epileptic Syndrome: A constellation of symptoms and signs, seizure types, etiology, anatomy, age of onset, precipitating factors, and other characteristics. Defining an epilepsy syndrome guides treatment and refines prognosis. Examples of epilepsy syndromes are Lennox-Gastaut, benign rolandic epilepsy, childhood absence epilepsy, juvenile myoclonic epilepsy, and West Syndrome.

Epileptic Twilight State: See Absence Status Epilepticus.

Febrile Seizures: Seizures that occur in 3 percent to 5 percent of children between the ages of 6 months and 5 years with fever *not* related to central nervous system (CNS) infection. Most occur during bacterial or viral infections between 18 and 24 months of age. Very few of these children develop epilepsy.

Febrile seizures can be divided into "simple" and "complex." (These adjectives have different meanings here than when applied to partial seizures!) Most children have "simple" febrile seizures. These convulsions last less than 15 minutes, lack focality, and do not recur within 24 hours.

Febrile seizures become "complex" when they exhibit one or more of the following features; last longer than 15 minutes, focal motor movements, a neurologic deficit, recur during the same day, or there is a parent or sibling with epilepsy. This differentiation is clinically useful because children with two or more "complex" features have a 6 percent risk of developing epilepsy by age 7, whereas children with simple febrile seizures have a less than 1 percent risk. In addition, children with complex febrile seizures need to be evaluated more aggressively for CNS infection or intracranial lesion.

Children with one or two simple febrile seizures do not require chronic antiepileptic drug therapy. These seizures appear to be a benign response to fever that is age related and later outgrown. Complex febrile seizures are more likely to require ongoing antiepileptic treatment.

Oral or rectal benzodiazepines may be useful for children with recurrent febrile seizures.

Fugue State (Poriomania): A prolonged period of aimless wandering with amnesia. Fugue states probably more often represent psychogenic dissociative disorders rather than postictal states.

Geschwind Syndrome: A cluster of personality traits thought over-represented in patients with temporal lobe epilepsy, particularly hypergraphia, hyperreligiosity, and hyposexuality. Other personality traits associated with temporal lobe epilepsy are; emotionality, manic tendencies, depression, humorlessness, anger, aggression, nascent philosophical interest, augmented sense of personal destiny, dependence, paranoia, moralism, guilt, obsessionalism, circumstantiality, and viscosity. (The prevalence of the Geschwind syndrome is still much debated.)

Grand Mal Seizures: Loosely translates from the French to "big bad" seizures. These are generalized tonic-clonic seizures or convulsions.

Grid: An array of electrodes placed on the surface of the brain to determine seizure onset or used to map cortical function such as speech.

Half-life: The time it takes for the serum concentration of an antiepileptic drug to decrease by 50 percent. Half-lives vary from as short as 5 hours for gabapentin to as long as 136 hours for phenobarbital (see Resources F and G). Metabolic rate affects serum half-lives. Consequently, hepatic induction will decrease the half-life of most AEDs, while decreased hepatic and renal function increase AED half-lives. (Half-lives tend to be increased in the elderly.)

When an AED with linear kinetics, such as phenobarbital, is discontinued, the serum level will decrease by 95 percent after five half-lives. Similarly, it takes five half-lives to reach a steady state when beginning a new AED. (Most AEDs exhibit linear kinetics, except for carbamazepine, phenytoin, and lamotrigine.)

Hemimegalencephaly: The affected side of the brain has a larger hemisphere and ventricle. The cortex is excessively thick with abnormal neuronal architecture. Giant neurons occur and calcifications may be seen in this rare developmental cerebral malformation.

Hemispherectomy: A type of epilepsy surgery reserved for patients with intractable epilepsy due to a globally dysfunctional hemisphere. Many of these patients already have a congenital hemiplegia opposite the affected hemisphere. During surgery, dysfunctional cortex is disconnected from the white matter and partially removed. In addition to excellent seizure control after this operation, many of these patients paradoxically have improvement in cognitive function.

Hertz: A unit of frequency (cycles per second) named after Heinrich Hertz, the discoverer of radio waves.

Heterotopia: A cluster of neurons in an abnormal location resulting from abnormal neuronal migration between the second and fifth months of gestation. Three major types of neuronal heterotopia are focal subcortical heterotopia, periventricular nodular heterotopia, and subcortical band heterotopia (double cortex syndrome). These misplaced neurons can be the source of epileptic seizures.

Hippocampal Sclerosis: Neuron loss and gliosis of the hippocampus associated with temporal lobe epilepsy. First described by Sommer in 1880, this distinctive pattern of cell loss can appear on magnetic resonance imaging as hippocampal atrophy and signal change.

Hyperekplexia (Startle Disease): An autosomal dominant movement disorder characterized by sudden loss of postural control related to a startle stimulus. Patients also may have spontaneous clonus. Symptoms may be confused with those of epilepsy.

Hypsarrhythmia: A dramatic pattern on the electroencephalogram in patients with infantile spasms. High voltage irregular slow waves, sharp waves, and multifocal epileptic spikes occur. Fast activity and burst suppression may also be seen.

Ictal: The period of clinical and electrical epileptic activity.

Impulsive Petit Mal (Juvenile Myoclonic Epilepsy of Janz): A primary generalized epilepsy with onset at age 12–18 years. Patients have myoclonic seizures, particularly when fatigued. These can occur in clusters and lead to convulsions. Absence seizures occur in up to a third of these patients. Response to valproate is excellent, but patients rarely outgrow this syndrome. Continued treatment is required.

Infantile Spasms: The first clinical description of infantile spasms appeared in the *Lancet* in 1841, provided by West describing these unusual seizures in his own son. Eighty-five percent of cases occur in infants before 12 months of age. Infantile spasms have a mortality of 10 percent to 20 percent and a morbidity of 75 percent to 90 percent. Approximately 25 percent of cases of infantile spasms evolve to Lennox-Gastaut syndrome. The best prognosis is seen in children who are normal when seizures begin and in whom no cause can be found for the spasms.

Seizures consist of flexor and/or extensor spasms of the body, which tend to occur in clusters. Infantile spasms are part of the triad of West's syndrome, which includes a hypsarrhythmic electroencephalogram and mental retardation. Up to 25 percent of cases of infantile spasms are associated with tuberous sclerosis.

Interictal: Refers to the time between seizures when patients are at their baseline.

Interictal Dysphoric Disorder: A recently described epilepsy specific affective disorder, with an intermittent and pleomorphic symptom profile. Patients exhibit three to eight of the following symptoms in the interictal period: depressive mood, anergia, pain, insomnia, fear, anxiety, paroxysmal irritability, and euphoric moods. Symptoms tend to be of sudden onset and brief duration. The most common are depressive mood, anergia, and irritability. Patients with temporal lobe epilepsy are at highest risk for interictal dysphoric syndrome.

Intractable Epilepsy: Seizures that persist despite appropriate treatment. Approximately 20 percent to 40 percent of patients have seizures that do not respond to adequate doses of appropriate antiepileptic drugs (AEDs). Usually, several AEDs are tried over a period of years before a patient is considered intractable. Patients with intractable epilepsy are potential candidates for investigational drug trials, epilepsy surgery, and novel treatments such as the vagal nerve stimulator.

Jamais Vu: A distortion of memory producing a feeling that a familiar experience has never occurred before (opposite of déjà vu.) Jamais vu and déjà vu are types of psychic auras and represent partial seizures.

Juvenile Absence Epilepsy: A primary generalized epilepsy occurring around puberty with absence seizures. Convulsions occur in approximately 50 percent of patients. Patients respond well to medication.

Juvenile Myoclonic Epilepsy of Janz: See Impulsive Petit Mal.

K complex: A normal feature of sleep architecture that appears in stage 2 of sleep. Sharp, slow, and fast components make up the K complex.

Kearns-Sayre Syndrome: A mitochondrial encephalomyopathy that occurs in children and is characterized by ophthalmoplegia and pigmentary retinopathy. Patients also may have ataxia, cardiac conduction block, elevated cerebrospinal fluid protein, and dementia. Unlike patients with myoclonic epilepsy and ragged red fibers or mitochondrial encephalomyopathy with lactic acidosis and strokelike episodes, only a few patients with Kearns-Sayre syndrome experience seizures.

Ketogenic Diet: Pioneered in the beginning of the 20th century, the ketogenic diet requires a high ratio of fat to carbohydrate and protein— typically 3:1 or 4:1—that produces systemic ketosis. Fluid also is restricted. Improvement in seizure control can occur when the diet is rigorously followed. The exact mechanism of action that promotes seizure control is not known.

Compliance may be a problem because of the strictness of the diet, care needed in meal preparation, and side effects of hunger and constipation. Nonetheless, the ketogenic diet is a reasonable treatment alternative for properly motivated patients and caregivers. In a Johns Hopkins study of 58 patients with mental retardation, cerebral palsy, and mixed seizure types, 29 percent became seizure-free and 38 percent had a better than 50 percent improvement. One third were not helped. In addition, 10 percent of the children discontinued their antiepileptic drugs.

Laminar Heterotopia: A neuronal migration disorder, also known as band heterotopia or double cortex syndrome. The sulcal pattern is normal, but an abnormal zone of gray matter is bordered on both sides by white matter. Appears restricted to females (see Heterotopia).

Landau-Kleffner Syndrome: A childhood syndrome of unknown etiology, consisting of progressive receptive and expressive aphasia, and an epileptiform electroencephalogram (EEG). Seventy percent of patients exhibit clinical seizures, most commonly partial complex. Epileptic activity is frequent on the EEG and tends to be more pronounced during sleep. Severe behavior problems commonly occur. Outcome is variable, with some children making a complete recovery as adults.

Lennox-Gastaut Syndrome: A childhood epileptic syndrome of intractable epilepsy, mental retardation, and slow spike and wave on the electroencephalogram. Multiple seizure types occur, particularly atypical absence, tonic, and atonic seizures. Myoclonic, partial and generalized tonic-clonic seizures also may be seen. Seizures are extremely difficult to control. Felbamate, lamotrigine, topiramate, valproate, and the benzodiazepines can reduce seizures. Oversedation with multiple medications is a frequent problem. The ketogenic diet may be helpful in reducing seizures. Lennox-Gastaut syndrome begins at ages 1–6 years and may evolve from West syndrome. In addition to the seizures, most of these children have other neurologic abnormalities. The prognosis is poor.

Lissencephaly: See Agyria.

Mental Retardation: Decreased intellectual functioning with an IQ less than 70, affecting language, visual, motor, and social abilities. One third of patients with severe mental retardation requiring institutionalization also have epilepsy.

Mesial Temporal Sclerosis: A specific pattern of neuronal cell loss, gliosis, and neuronal reorganization in the medial temporal lobe commonly responsible for partial complex seizures. The hippocampal atrophy of mesial temporal sclerosis can often be detected by magnetic resonance imaging. Many patients give a history of febrile seizures. Patients with intractable epilepsy due to mesial temporal sclerosis can be cured by temporal lobectomy 80 percent to 90 percent of the time.

Mitochondrial Encephalomyopathy with Lactic Acidosis and Stroke-like Episodes: A maternally inherited syndrome characterized by normal early development, recurrent headaches, and vomiting. Patients suffer strokelike episodes and almost always have seizures. Ataxia, dementia, exercise intolerance, muscle weakness, myoclonus, sensorineural hearing loss, and short stature may be present. (Patients may resemble those with myoclonic epilepsy and ragged-red fibers.)

Monotherapy: The treatment of epilepsy with a single medication rather than a combination. Monotherapy has distinct advantages over polytherapy in many patients, including absence of drug-drug interactions, fewer side effects, simpler dosing, and lower cost. However, not all patients can be controlled with monotherapy.

Myoclonic Epilepsy with Ragged-Red Fibers: Previously described by Ramsey Hunt as dyssynergia cerebellaris myoclonica, myoclonic epilepsy with ragged-red fibers (MERRF) is the first hereditary epilepsy syndrome to be characterized by a specific mitochondrial mutation. MERRF is a maternally inherited syndrome characterized by ataxia, myoclonus, and seizures. Patients may also have deafness, dementia, lactic acidosis, lipomas, peripheral neuropathy, and short stature. Muscle biopsy reveals ragged red fibers, which are related to subsarcolemmal mitochondrial accumulations in muscle fibers. All patients with MERRF have seizures.

Myoclonus: Brief motor jerks that may represent epileptic seizures or nonepileptic etiologies. A history of myoclonus can help point to a specific epilepsy syndrome, such as myoclonic epilepsy of Janz.

Neuronal Migration Disorders: Cerebral malformations such as focal cortical dysplasia, polymicrogyria, and the nodular heterotopias occur when migrating neurons do not reach their appropriate cortical destinations. Genetic factors and a variety of intrauterine insults such as drugs, infections, radiation, and/or toxins may be responsible.

Nonconvulsive Status Epilepticus: A prolonged seizure state characterized by mental slowness, confusion, or even stupor or coma. Nonconvulsive status epilepticus may be due to either persistent absence seizures or partial complex seizures. An electroencephalogram will be necessary to confirm this diagnosis.

Nonepileptic Seizures (Pseudoseizures, Psychogenic Seizures): These may be physiologic events such as syncope, tics, or transient ischemic attacks that are mistaken as epileptic seizures. More commonly, staring spells, abnormal movements, or convulsions result from psychiatric problems such as conversion disorder, malingering, or panic attacks. The diagnosis of recurrent unexplained spells can be very difficult to make with only the patient as witness. Consequently, video-EEG may be required in order to diagnose nonepileptic seizures.

Pachygryria: A type of cortical dysplasia with wide cortical convolutions and heterotopic neurons.

Partial Seizure: A seizure that begins in a specific cortical location, or focus. An anatomic abnormality, such as a brain tumor or an arteriovenous malformation, or an electrical lesion that can only be seen by electroencephalography may be responsible. Partial seizures are divided into "simple" and "complex" seizures. Consciousness is preserved in partial simple seizures but altered in partial complex seizures. Partial seizures are the most common seizure type in adults.

Partial Complex Seizure: A partial complex seizure begins in a specific location, such as the temporal or frontal lobe, and causes alteration of consciousness. Temporal lobe partial complex seizures are sometimes called psychomotor seizures. Typically, these last from 30 seconds to several minutes. Automatisms, such as lip smacking, chewing, swallowing, and fumbling with clothes, commonly occur. Because of the alteration of consciousness, patients may not always be aware they have had a seizure. This limits their ability to self-report seizure frequency and underlines the importance of a witness or caretaker to assist in medical management.

Partial Simple Seizure: A partial simple seizure begins in a specific brain location and does not cause alteration of consciousness. For example, a seizure that begins in the frontal lobe and causes motor movements of the opposite extremity is a partial simple seizure. An epileptic aura, such as a smell, visual hallucination, or sound, is also a partial simple seizure. Partial simple seizures may be self-limited or evolve into partial complex or secondarily generalized seizures.

Petit Mal Seizure: See Childhood Absence Epilepsy.

Petit Mal Variant: A slow spike and wave pattern seen on the electroencephalogram at 1–2.5 Hertz. This pattern differs from the three Hertz pattern seen in classic "petit mal" absence seizures. Petit mal variant is seen in Lennox-Gastaut syndrome, a severe type of childhood epilepsy.

Pharmacodynamic Interactions: The physiologic consequence of combining drugs with similar mechanisms of action. The results may be additive, more than additive, or antagonistic.

Pharmacokinetic Interactions: One drug can alter serum concentrations of another. Several types of pharmacokinetic interactions occur, including effects on drug distribution, metabolism, and excretion. Enzyme inhibition or induction by one drug often affects the half-life of another. For example, valproate extends the half-life of lamotrigine, whereas carbamazepine decreases the half-life of topiramate. Pharmacokinetic interactions can be assessed directly by measuring antiepileptic drug levels.

Polycystic Ovary Syndrome: Characterized by polycystic ovaries, hirsutism, acne, obesity, elevated androgens, an elevated luteinizing hormone (LH):follicle stimulating hormone (FSH) ratio, chronic anovulation, and insulin resistance. Polycystic ovary syndrome is increased in women with temporal lobe epilepsy fourfold over that of women in the general population. In addition, women taking sodium valproate have been found to have an increase in polycystic ovary syndrome, but the relationship to the drug remains under investigation.

Polymicrogyria: A cortical abnormality with excessive numbers of small gyri. Polymicrogyria can be focal or diffuse. Intrauterine cytomegalovirus infection can cause polymicrogyria. Ischemia may also be responsible. Congenital bilateral perisylvian syndrome due to polymicrogyria consists of developmental delay, pseudobulbar paresis, and typical imaging findings. Most patients have seizures.

Polypharmacology: Multiple actions of a single drug. For example, topiramate limits sustained repetitive firing via state-dependent blockade of sodium channels, potentiates GABA-mediated neuroinhibition at GABA (A) sites, blocks glutamate-mediated neuroexcitation, and is a carbonic anhydrase inhibitor.

Polytherapy: The treatment of epilepsy with medication combinations. Because not all patients can be controlled with monotherapy, sometimes two or more medications are effective. Whenever possible, drugs with complementary mechanisms of action and different side-effect profiles should be used. For example, phenytoin and valproate represent a logical combination, whereas phenobarbital and primidone would offer more additive side effects than therapeutic advantages.

Poriomania: See Fugue State.

Positron Emission Tomography: A computerized imaging technique that allows imaging of cerebral metabolic rates, receptor densities, and blood flow. Most commonly, radioactive labeled F-fluoro-2-deoxyglucose assesses cerebral glucose metabolism. During the interictal period, positron emission tomography (PET) scans often identify regions of cerebral hypometabolism that correlate with the epileptogenic zone.

During a seizure, this same region becomes hypermetabolic. PET may reveal abnormal brain regions not seen on magnetic resonance imaging.

Postictal Psychosis: Psychosis in epilepsy can occur in the interictal, ictal, and postictal state. Although interictal psychosis is the most frequent type of psychosis, postictal psychosis comprises 25 percent of the psychoses in this population.

Postictal psychosis usually occurs after a cluster of convulsions. A lucid interval lasting 1 to 6 days frequently precedes the psychosis. Most patients exhibit abnormal mood and paranoid delusions. Psychotic episodes last days to weeks. Neuroleptic treatment may not be required. Postictal psychosis may be related to increased dopamine release.

Prolactin: A hormone produced by the anterior pituitary gland. Serum prolactin levels often increase 3 to 20 times baseline after a seizure. Prolactin levels peak 10 to 20 minutes after a seizure and return to baseline in an hour. Prolactin levels are used along with the electroencephalogram to help differentiate epileptic seizures from nonepileptic spells. Because prolactin levels vary during the day, a repeat serum prolactin level 24 hours later is needed for comparison. Prolactin elevations occur in 90 percent of tonic-clonic seizures, approximately 70 percent of partial complex seizures, and 10 percent of partial simple seizures. Consequently, the absence of a prolactin rise is less helpful than a definite increase. Prolactin usually does not increase in frontal lobe partial complex seizures. Prolactin elevations also can occur from many other sources, including pregnancy, prolactinomas, general anesthesia, phenothiazines, butyrophenones, and metoclopramide.

Pseudoseizures: See Nonepileptic Seizures.

Psychomotor Variant: An electroencephalographic pattern, composed of rhythmic bursts of theta waves, that resembles an epileptic discharge. Most often seen in drowsiness, this normal variant is also known as "rhythmic midtemporal discharges" or "rhythmic temporal theta bursts."

Psychomotor Epilepsy: A historical term referring to the varied psychic phenomena that occur during certain types of seizures. The vast majority of seizures of this type originate in the temporal lobe. Seizures beginning in the temporal lobe may cause autonomic, dysmnesic, emotional, gustatory, olfactory, visual, and other strange symptoms.

Pyknolepsy: An older term for childhood absence epilepsy.

Radioligand: A radioactive pharmaceutical tracer used in positron emission tomography or single photon emission computed tomography. Radioligands can be fabricated to evaluate glucose or oxygen utilization, cerebral blood flow, benzodiazepine, cholinergic, or opiate receptor distribution, and other aspects of the central nervous system.

Rasmussen's Encephalitis: Usually presenting in children, Rasmussen's encephalitis is characterized by progressive hemiplegia, mental decline, and intractable seizures. About 50 percent of patients manifest epilepsia partialis continua. Brain biopsy reveals cortical inflammation with gliosis and tissue destruction. Traditional treatment has been functional hemispherectomy. The benefits of plasma exchange and immunosuppressant treatment are under evaluation for this probable autoimmune disorder.

Schizencephaly: A developmental abnormality resulting in a cleft extending from the pial cerebral surface to the ependymal surface of the ventricle. Dysplastic gray matter often lines the cleft. Heterotopias may be present. Patients with schizencephaly may have severe developmental delay, microcephaly, and seizures.

Sharp Wave: A sharply contoured wave on the EEG too prolonged to meet spike criteria, but may suggest epileptic activity. Sharp waves last between 70 and 200 milliseconds.

Single Photon Emission Computed Tomography: Noninvasive nuclear medicine imaging of cerebral blood flow used at epilepsy centers to help determine the lateralization and localization of a seizure focus. When the radioligand is injected at the onset of a seizure, single photon emission computed tomography (SPECT) scans can reveal cerebral hyperperfusion at the seizure focus. In between seizures (interictally), this same region may be hypoperfused.

Ictal SPECT reliably identifies the seizure focus in temporal lobe epilepsy more than 90 percent of the time. Ictal SPECT can also provide useful localization information in extratemporal epilepsy.

Whereas traditional positron emission tomography (PET) measures cerebral glucose metabolism, SPECT measures cerebral blood flow. Both tests are complementary in the presurgical evaluation of the intractable epilepsy patient.

Spike: A specific electroencephalogram abnormality associated with epileptic seizures. A spike must last 20–70 milliseconds, display a pointed peak, and be distinct from the background.

Spike Wave Stupor: See Absence Status Epilepticus.

Startle Disease: See Hyperekplexia.

Status Epilepticus: Recurrent or persistent seizures that create a fixed and lasting epileptic condition. Status epilepticus requires immediate evaluation for its underlying cause and simultaneous treatment of the seizures (see Resource S). Status epilepticus can be life-threatening, with mortality ranging from 1 percent to 10 percent. Any seizure or cluster of seizures without recovery that lasts 30 minutes or more qualifies as status epilepticus. (Therapeutic intervention should be attempted long before, however.)

Strip: A single row of electrical contacts used for monitoring electrical brain activity directly from the cortex. Strips can be placed through a burr hole or after craniotomy.

Sturge-Weber Syndrome (Encephalofacial Angiomatosis): A neurocutaneous syndrome of uncertain inheritance. The constellation of facial nevus, mental retardation, contralateral hemiparesis, and glaucoma characterizes this syndrome. More than 70 percent of patients develop epilepsy, typically beginning in childhood. Status epilepticus often occurs. Patients have leptomeningeal angiomatosis and develop intracranial calcifications. Seizures may be refractory to antiepileptic drug therapy, although some patients dramatically improve with surgical resection.

Subacute Sclerosing Panencephalitis: A rare progressive encephalopathy resulting from exposure to measles. Intellectual deterioration, personality changes, and intractable myoclonus occur. A characteristic suppression-burst pattern occurs on the EEG in 80 percent of patients.

Subclinical Seizures (Electrographic Seizures): These seizures are visible on the EEG, but the patient does not exhibit clinical symptoms. Electroencephalography often detects subclinical seizures during sleep.

Subclinical Rhythmic Electrographic Discharge of Adults: Rhythmic slowing of the temporo-parieto-occipital junction seen in some adults, which may be associated with aging or cerebrovascular disease. Rhythmic, subclinical rhythmic electrographic discharge of adults (SREDA) does not indicate seizure activity and is a normal variant.

Subdural Electrodes: These electrodes are small metal contacts imbedded in silastic in different configurations, either strips or grids (see Grids). They are placed on the cerebral cortex to record electrical activity and assist in the localization of the seizure focus. Subdural electrodes can also be used as stimulation contacts in speech or other brain mapping.

Temporal Lobectomy: A surgical procedure pioneered by neurosurgeon Dr. Wilder Penfield for the cure of epilepsy related to temporal lobe seizures. Patients with mesial temporal sclerosis respond exceptionally well to temporal lobectomy.

Therapeutic Range: Measured serum concentrations of antiepileptic drugs within which most patients have good antiepileptic effect with minimal toxicity. For example, the therapeutic range of carbamazepine is 4–12 µg/ml, phenytoin 10–20 µg/ml, and valproate 50–150 µg/ml. (See Resource F.)

Note, however, that many patients have good medication results with serum levels lower or higher than the published therapeutic range, while some patients experience toxicity within that range. Consequently, these measurements provide a *guideline* for treatment and constitute only one component of the clinical picture. Doses should not be changed merely because of a serum level lower or higher than the therapeutic range.

In addition, serum levels vary depending on the timing of the sample relative to the last dose, particularly for AEDs with shorter half-lives.

Reasons to measure serum AED levels include:

1. A new AED has been added
2. Patient appears toxic
3. Uncontrolled seizures
4. Compliance is suspect

Tonic: Stiffening of flexor or extensor muscles during a seizure. May occur as a tonic seizure or part of a tonic-clonic seizure.

Tuberous Sclerosis: Accounts for 25 percent of cases of infantile spasms. Half of all patients with tuberous sclerosis (TS) and seizures present with infantile spasms. The prevalence of epilepsy in TS has been measured at greater than 80 percent.

Inheritance is autosomal dominant, giving a 50 percent chance of inheritance to the child of one affected parent. Parents may be so mildly affected that they are unaware of the disease. I have seen a number of adults with mild seizure disorders who did not know they had tuberous sclerosis. The diagnosis is essential for genetic counseling. Children may be more severely affected than their parents. In addition, TS occurs by spontaneous mutation 60 percent of the time.

Learning disability is common and, when severe, is usually accompanied by seizures. Clinical features of the syndrome are achromic nevi, adenoma sebaceum, subungual fibromas, shagreen patches, cardiac rhabdomyomas, renal tumors, and retinal phacomas. Cortical tubers, calcified hamartomas, and rare intraventricular giant cell astrocytomas occur. Patients should have cardiac and renal ultrasounds and an ophthalmologic exam to screen for extraneurologic manifestations.

Uncinate Fits: Partial seizures from the anterior mesial temporal lobe or orbital frontal structures characterized by olfactory symptoms. Typically, the abnormal smell is unpleasant, often described as "burnt rubber." These seizures have traditionally been associated with neoplasms.

Vagal Nerve Stimulator (Neurocybernetic Prosthesis): The first implantable device approved by the U.S. Food and Drug Administration for seizure control. A battery powered programmable generator, similar to a cardiac pacemaker, sends repeated stimulation via an electrode attached to the left vagus nerve. Many patients experience significant seizure reduction.

Version: The turning of head and eyes during a seizure. Sustained versive movements usually indicate a contralateral seizure focus from the frontal, temporal, or occipital lobes.

Vertex Sharp Wave: A normal feature of drowsiness and light sleep. Vertex sharp waves should not be confused with epileptic spikes.

Wada: Also known as intracarotid Amytal procedure. Pioneered by Juhn Wada, this test evaluates memory and laterality of language before temporal lobectomy. A carotid angiogram is performed, followed by an anesthetic injection. While one hemisphere is anesthetized, the other is assessed for memory and language function. After the patient recovers, the procedure is repeated on the other hemisphere.

Surgical candidates must demonstrate sufficient memory ability in the temporal lobe that will remain after surgery. Identification of language laterality allows the neurosurgeon to tailor the operation of the temporal cortex to protect language function.

West Syndrome: A triad of infantile spasms, mental retardation, and a hypsarrhythmic electroencephalogram. Most cases occur between the ages of 3 and 7 months, with a prevalence of 0.3 per 1,000. Treatment of the seizures is with ACTH or antiepileptics such as valproate and the benzodiazepines. Felbamate, lamotrigine, topiramate, and vigabatrin can also help control infantile spasms. Only about 5 percent of patients have a normal outcome.

Bibliography

Selected Bibliography

1. Engel J, Pedley T (eds.). *Epilepsy: A Comprehensive Textbook*, Vols. 1–3. Philadelphia: Lippincott-Raven, 1997.
2. Fisher R (ed.). *Imitators of Epilepsy*. New York: Demos, 1994.
3. Freeman J, Freeman J, Kelly M. *The Ketogenic Diet: A Treatment for Epilepsy,* 3rd ed. New York: Demos, 2000.
4. Kaplan P, Louiseau P, Fisher R, Jallon P. *Epilepsy A to Z: A Glossary of Epilepsy Terminology.* New York: Demos, 1995.
5. Petersdorf R, et al. (eds.). *Harrison's Principles of Internal Medicine.* New York: McGraw-Hill, 1983.
6. Porter R et al. (eds.). *Alcohol and Seizures.* Philadelphia: FA Davis, 1990.
7. Wilner A. *Epilepsy: 199 Answers.* New York: Demos, 1996.
8. Wyllie E (ed.). *The Treatment of Epilepsy: Principles and Practice.* Philadelphia: Lea & Febiger, 1993.

More Epilepsy Books of Interest

1. Buckel M, Buckel T. *Mom, I Have a Staring Problem.* Brandenton: Marian Buckel, 1992.
2. Davidson A. *Embrace the Dawn: One Woman's Story of Triumph over Epilepsy,* McCall: Sylvan Creek Press, 1989.
3. Devinsky O. *A Guide to Understanding and Living with Epilepsy.* Philadelphia: FA Davis, 1994.

4. Fishman S. *A Bomb in the Brain: A Heroic Tale of Science, Surgery, and Survival.* New York: Avon Books, 1988.
5. Freeman J, Vining E, Pillas D. *Seizures and Epilepsy in Childhood: A Guide for Parents.* Baltimore: Johns Hopkins University Press, 1991.
6. Goss S (ed.). *Epilepsy: I Can Live With That!* Epilepsy Foundation of Victoria, Inc., 1995.
7. Gumnit R. *Living Well with Epilepsy*, 2nd ed. New York: Demos, 1996.
8. Gumnit R. *Your Child and Epilepsy.* New York: Demos, 1995.
9. Heymann, J. *Equal Partners.* Boston: Little, Brown, 1995.
10. Richard A, Reiter J. *Epilepsy: A New Approach.* New York: Walker and Company, 1995.
11. Santilli N. *Managing Seizure Disorders.* Philadelphia: Lippincott-Raven, 1996.
12. Schachter S (ed.). *Brainstorms: Epilepsy in Our Words.* New York: Raven Press, 1993.
13. Schachter S (ed.). *The Brainstorms Companion.* New York: Raven Press, 1995.
14. Schachter S, Montouris G, Pellock J. *The Brainstorms Family, Epilepsy on Our Terms.* Philadelphia: Lippincott-Raven, 1996.
15. Schachter S, Rowan A (eds.). *The Brainstorms Healer, Epilepsy in Our Experience.* Philadelphia: Lippincott-Raven, 1998.

Index

Abnormal neurologic examinations, 31
Absence epilepsy/absence seizures, 36,
   40, 45, 54, 126, 127, 163, 231, 232,
   233, 238, 239, 244
   as first seizure, differential diagnosis of
     epilepsy and, 10
   intractable epilepsy and, 15
   nonepileptic seizures vs., 111
   during pregnancy, 48
   status epilepticus, 102, 231, 236,
     245
Abuse as child, 6
Acetazolamide (Diamox), 35–36
   adverse effect of phenytoin/
     carbamazepine levels and, 141
   intractable epilepsy and, 13
   ketogenic diet treatment and, 24
   mechanisms of action of, 134
Acidosis in pregnancy, 48
Acquired epileptic aphasia (Landau-
   Kleffner syndrome), 126
Acronyms list, 228–230
Acupuncture alternative therapy, 123
Adapting to life post-surgery, 20–21
Adenosine receptors, 46
Adolescent onset (*See also* Childhood
   epilepsy), 31
Adrenocorticotropic hormone (ACTH) as
   alternative therapy, 121
Adult onset epilepsy, 1–11
Age and epilepsy, 163

first seizure and differential diagnosis
   of epilepsy, 2–3
vs. side effects in AEDs, 41
Aggressive behavior, 13, 58
Agranulocytosis and AEDs, 40, 41
Agyria, 231
Aicardi syndrome, 231
Alcohol use/abuse, 25, 26, 27, 28, 36, 58,
   68, 71, 85–93, 126
AEDs and, 90–91, 92–93
   alcohol-related seizures and, 86–87
   aneurysms and, 89
   barbiturates and, 93
   blood chemistry levels in, 86
   carbamazepine and, 93
   CAT scan as diagnostic tool in, 86
   confusion in, 88
   delirium tremens and, 85, 86
   detoxification and, 85
   diazepam and, 85, 88, 91–92
   drug abuse and, 87
   EEG results in, 86, 89–90
   fosphenytoin (Cerebyx) and, 90
   head injury and, 88, 91
   heavy drinking and, increased seizure
     activity and, 92
   hepatic failure in, 93
   hypertension in, 87
   hypoalbuminemia in, 93
   hypoglycemia and, 87
   hypomagnesemia in, 87